Self-assessment for the MRCP Part 2 Written Paper:
Volume 2 Case Histories

Self-assessment for the MRCP Part 2 Written Paper:
Volume 2
Case Histories

Narinder Bajaj MA MRCP PhD
Honorary Lecturer in Neurology
Specialist Registrar in Neurology
National Hospital for Neurology
London

Balwinder Bajaj BSc MRCP PhD
Consultant Physician and Cardiologist
The Royal Oldham Hospital
Oldham

Karim Meeran MD FRCP
Consultant Endocrinologist
Charing Cross and Hammersmith Hospitals
London

EDITORIAL ADVISOR

Huw Benyon BSc MD FRCP
Consultant Physician and Rheumatologist
The Royal Free Hospital School of Medicine
Royal Free Hospital
London

Blackwell
Science

© 2002 by Blackwell Science Ltd
a Blackwell Publishing Company
Editorial Offices:
Osney Mead, Oxford OX2 0EL, UK
  Tel: +44 (0)1865 206206
108 Cowley Road, Oxford OX4 1JF, UK
  Tel: +44 (0)1865 791100
Blackwell Publishing USA, 350 Main Street, Malden, MA 02148-5018, USA
  Tel: +1 781 388 8250
Iowa State Press, a Blackwell Publishing Company, 2121 State Avenue, Ames, Iowa 50014-8300, USA
  Tel: +1 515 292 0140
Blackwell Munksgaard, Nørre Søgade 35, PO Box 2148, Copenhagen, DK-1016, Denmark
  Tel: +45 77 33 33 33
Blackwell Publishing Asia, 54 University Street, Carlton, Victoria 3053, Australia
  Tel: +61 (0)3 9347 0300
Blackwell Verlag, Kurfürstendamm 57, 10707 Berlin, Germany
  Tel: +49 (0)30 32 79 060
Blackwell Publishing, 10 rue Casimir Delavigne, 75006 Paris, France
  Tel: +33 1 53 10 33 10

First published 2002
Reprinted 2003

Catalogue records for this title are available from the Library of Congress and the British Library

ISBN 0-632-06441-2

Set in 8/10 Frutiger Condensed by Best-set Typesetter Ltd., Hong Kong
Printed and bound in Great Britain by MPG Books Ltd, Bodmin Cornwall

For further information on Blackwell Science, visit our website:
www.blackwell-science.com

Contents

Preface

This book is part of a series of three, designed to provide a revision course for the written part of the MRCP examination. Together with Volume 1 (Picture Tests) and Volume 3 (Data Interpretation), they comprise a significant volume of work, giving ample coverage of the MRCP syllabus.

The 60 case histories contained in this volume cover the medical topics most amenable to grey case presentation. Subjects more amenable to data interpretation are covered in Volume 3; thus these two volumes are designed to be used together to provide full coverage of the syllabus. There is a strong emphasis on the candidate being able to provide the most likely answer as well as a differential diagnosis. This is to encourage skills transferable from textbook learning to the actual clinical situation. The answers to these case histories are graded (from three stars for the preferred answer) to reflect this.

The writing of this text has been a lengthy one and we would like to thank all members of our respective families for their support and patience during this time. NPSB and BPSB would especially like to thank their father (a long established author) for his words of wisdom.

NPSB, BPSB, KM 2001.

Normal values

Chemical pathology

Sodium (Na)	135–145 mmol/l
Potassium (K)	3.5–5.0 mmol/l
Urea (U)	3.3–6.7 mmol/l
Creatinine (Cr)	45–120 µmol/l
Bicarbonate (HCO_3^-)	22–30 mmol/l
Calcium (Ca)	2.2–2.67 mmol/l
Phosphate (PO_4)	0.8–1.5 mmol/l
Magnesium (Mg)	0.7–1.1 mmol/l
Copper (Cu)	11–22 µmol/l
Caeruloplasmin	0.20–0.60 g/l
Chloride (Cl)	95–105 mmol/l
Cholesterol (Ch)	3.6–7.8 mmol/l
Triglyceride (TG)	0.8–2.1 mmol/l
Creatinine phosphokinase (CPK)	
Male	17–148 IU/l
Female	10–79 IU/l
Urate	180–420 µmol/l
Glucose (fasting)	4.5–5.8 mmol/l
Glycosylated haemoglobin (HbA_{1c})	3.8–6.4%
Lactate	0.6–1.8 mmol/l
Total protein (TP)	60–80 g/l
Albumin (Alb)	35–50 g/l
Bilirubin (Bili)	3–20 µmol/l
Alkaline phosphatase (Alk P)	30–130 IU/l
Alanine amino transferase (ALT)	5–30 IU/l
Aspartate transaminase (AST)	10–50 IU/l
Gamma glutamyl transferase (GGT)	5–40 IU/l
Amylase	46–330 IU/l
Globulin (Glob)	25–35 g/l
Alphafetoprotein	<10 IU/ml
Angiotensin-converting enzyme	204–358 U/l
Plasma osmolality	275–295 mosmol/l

Endocrine tests

Total serum thyroxine (T4)	58–174 nmol/l
Total serum triiodothyronine (T3)	1.2–3.1 nmol/l
Free serum thyroxine (FT4)	13–30 pmol/l
Free triiodothyronine (FT3)	2.8–7.1 pmol/l
Thyroid stimulating hormone (TSH)	0.3–6.0 mU/l
Testosterone	
Male	9–35 nmol/l
Female	0.9–3.1 nmol/l

Cortisol
  (0900 hours)   280–700 nmol/l
  (2400 hours)   80–280 nmol/l

Prolactin
  Male   <450 mU/l
  Female   <600 mU/l
Adrenocorticotrophic hormone (ACTH)   <10–80 ng/l
Growth hormone (GH)   <20 mU/l (<5 ng/ml after 75 g
                                  oral glucose challenge)

Urinary values

Urine copper	15–78 µmol/24 h (0.01–0.06 mg/24 h)
Urine vanillyl mandelic acid (VMA)	5–35 µmol/24 h
Urine creatinine	0.13–0.22 mmol/kg body weight, daily
Urine protein (quantitative)	<0.15 g/24 h
Urine sodium	50–125 mmol/l
	100–250 mmol/24 h

Blood gas measurements (room air)

pO_2	11.2–14 kPa
pCO_2	4.6–6.0 kPa
pH	7.35–7.45
Base excess	0 ± 2 mmol/l

Haematology

Haemoglobin (Hb)	
Male	13–18 g/dl
Female	11.5–15 g/dl
White cell count (WCC)	$4.0–11.0 \times 10^9$/l
Red cell count (RBC)	$3.8–5.8 \times 10^{12}$/l
Packed cell volume (PCV) (haematocrit)	
Male	0.4–0.54
Female	0.37–0.47
Mean corpuscular volume (MCV)	79.0–96.0 fl
Mean corpuscular haemoglobin (MCH)	27.0–32.0 pg
Mean corpuscular haemoglobin concentration (MCHC)	31.5–36.0 g/dl
Platelet (Plt)	$150–450 \times 10^9$/l
Reticulocyte count	0.2–2%
Prothrombin time (PT)	12–16 s
International normalized ratio (INR)	0.90–1.20
Activated partial thromboplastin time (APTT)	23–33 s
Thrombin time (TT)	15–19 s
Fibrinogen	1.5–4.5 g/l

Vitamin B_{12}	180–1100 ng/l (150–675 pmol/l)
Folate (serum)	4.0–18.0 µg/l (5–63 nmol/l)
Folate (red cell)	160–640 µg/l
Iron (Fe)	13–32 µmol/l (50–150 µg/dl)
Iron binding capacity (TIBC)	40–80 µmol/l (250–410 µg/dl)
Ferritin	15–250 µg/l (5.8–120 nmol/l)
Transferrin	1.2–2 g/l
Neutrophils	$2.50–7.50 \times 10^9$/l
Lymphocytes	$1.30–4.00 \times 10^9$/l
Monocytes	$0.0–1.00 \times 10^9$/l
Eosinophils	$0.04–0.40 \times 10^9$/l
Basophils	$0.0–0.10 \times 10^9$/l

Erythrocyte sedimentation rate

Male	age/2 mm/h
Female	age + 10/2 mm/h

Immunology

Immunoglobulin G (IGG)	7.0–18.6 g/l
Immunoglobulin M (IGM)	0.49–2.0 g/l
Immunoglobulin A (IGA)	0.78–4.8 g/l
Anti-double stranded DNA titre (dsDNA)	<60 IU/ml
Anti-mitochondrial antibody	10–47 µmol/l
Complement (C3)	0.55–1.30 g/l
Complement (C4)	0.20–0.60 g/l
C-reactive protein	<10 mg/l

Cerebrospinal fluid

Protein	0.15–0.4 g/l
Glucose	2.8–4.5 g/l
Cells	<5 white/red cells mm^{-3}
Pressure	70–180 mm H_2O

Haemodynamic normal values
(pressure measurements in mmHg)

Systemic arterial

Peak systolic/end-diastolic	100–140/60–90
Mean	70–105

Left ventricular

Peak systolic/end diastolic	100–140/3–12

Left atrial (or pulmonary capillary wedge)

Mean	2–12
a wave	3–10
v wave	3–15

Pulmonary artery

Peak systolic/end diastolic	15–30/4–14
Mean	9–17

Right ventricular

Peak systolic/end diastolic	15–30/2–7

Right atrial

Mean	2–6
a wave	2–8
v wave	2–7

Resistances [(dyn.s)/cm^5]

Systemic vascular resistance	700–1600
Total pulmonary resistance	100–300
Pulmonary vascular resistance	30–130

Flows

Cardiac index (l/min m^{-2})	2.4–3.8
Stroke index (mm/beat m^{-2})	30–65

A 68-year-old printer specializing in the use of lead blocks was seen in casualty having difficulty walking. His wife said his problems had started 4 months earlier, when he became increasingly absent-minded and forgetful. He believed strangers were in the house stealing his possessions and although he felt their presence he denied ever seeing them. A medical friend of the family thought he was becoming schizophrenic and gave him a supply of trifluoperazine tablets to calm him down.

On examination, he had a mask-like facies and a staring gaze. Glabellar tap was positive. He had bilateral cogwheeling rigidity in the upper limb. His gait was festinant and his postural reflexes were impaired. Mental test scores were low, owing to a poor concentration span and an impaired short-term memory. He had a postural drop of 30 mmHg when standing.

A Give the likely diagnosis.

B What would be your initial management and what tests would you request?

A Diffuse (or cortical) Lewy body disease (DLBD) with dementia. **✳✳✳**
Multiple system atrophy type A (MSA type A). **✳✳**
Dementia, e.g. due to chronic lead poisoning with extra-pyramidal side-effects caused by
trifluoperazine. **✳**

The history here is of an elderly man with a dementing condition with marked paranoid delusions, as
well as an extra-pyramidal picture and a postural drop. The latter is perhaps due to an autonomic
neuropathy, although both this and the parkinsonism may have been caused by the major tranquillizer.
    DLBD with dementia is a post-mortem diagnosis and has become an increasingly recognized
condition. In this case it would explain the dementia, the parkinsonism and the autonomic failure.
Paranoid delusions are said to be characteristic of DLBD.
    MSA type A (previously known as Shy–Drager syndrome), comprising idiopathic parkinsonism with
marked autonomic failure, could also be a possibility. The characteristic pathological lesion of MSA is
the glial cytoplasmic inclusion; widespread cell loss and gliosis are seen in multiple areas of the brain.
The presence of dementia makes this diagnosis less likely as there is relative cognitive sparing. Both of
the above conditions are poorly responsive to L-dopa.

Chronic lead poisoning in the adult has a variety of features:
Haematological. Haemolytic anaemia with basophilic stippling due to inhibition of haem synthesis.
Neurological. Motor neuropathy, neuropsychiatric sequelae or a 'subclinical' drop in I.Q.
Renal. Tubular dysfunction causing, for example, gouty nephropathy.
Other. Arthropathy, gout.
Gastrointestinal. e.g. constipation and a blue line around the gums due to sulphide deposition.

B Stop the trifluoperazine. **✳✳✳**
Consider using an atypical neuroleptic agent, e.g. olanzapine or clozapine. **✳✳**
Consider an L-dopa challenge. **✳✳**
Treat postural hypotension with elasticated stockings, a high salt diet, head-up tilt of the bed at night,
fludrocortisone ± ephedrine, and DDAVP. **✳✳**

Request:

Blood film for basophilic stippling and serum lead level
CT scanning: this will be normal in idiopathic parkinsonism but may show cerebellar or brain-stem
    atrophy in MSA.
MRI: this can be normal in idiopathic parkinsonism, MSA and DLBD. However, MRI may show an
    altered putaminal signal in MSA with a low T2-weighted signal change due to iron deposition and a
    high T2-lateral putaminal signal. Brain-stem or cerebellar atrophy may also be seen in MSA.
    Cortical atrophy may be visible in DLBD.
Fluoridopa positron emission tomography (PET): this may show decreased striatal uptake in idiopathic
    parkinsonism or MSA and decreased caudate uptake in MSA.
Anal sphincter EMG.
Autonomic function testing.
Neuropsychometric testing.

A middle-aged woman was admitted via the casualty department, confused and unkempt. She had been found by a neighbour on the floor of her bed-sit. The medications brought with her were spironolactone and ferrous sulphate. On admission she resisted all attempts at examination. A cursory examination established that she was afebrile, with a grossly distended, non-tender abdomen that also demonstrated shifting dullness.

The results of her initial investigations were as follows:
Hb 12.4 g/dl, WCC 6×10^9/l, Plts 171×10^9/l, MCV 112 fl, MCH 37 pg,
Blood film: target cells, acanthocytes,
PT 18.7 s.

Sodium 126 mmol/l, potassium 6.4 mmol/l, bicarbonate 20 mmol/l, urea 14 mmol/l, creatinine 150 μmol/l, random blood glucose 4.4 mmol/l, bilirubin 73 μmol/l, alkaline phosphatase 98 IU/l, AST 40 IU/l, ALT 26 IU/l, total protein 80 g/l, albumin 27 g/l, globulins 53 g/l, GGT 44 IU/l.

A What is the most likely underlying basis for the confusion?

B What tests and physical signs would help to confirm your diagnosis?

C How would you manage this patient?

A Hepatic encephalopathy. ✲✲✲
Infection. ✲✲
Wernicke–Korsakoff encephalopathy. ✲
Hyponatraemic encephalopathy. ✲

B Hepatic flap. ✲✲✲
EEG. ✲✲
Ammonia level. ✲✲
Inability to draw a 5-pointed star. ✲

C Use lactulose and neomycin to encourage bowel-emptying and reduce the protein load produced by the bowel flora.
　Prescribe a low-protein diet and thiamine supplements.
　An ascitic tap (with fluid sent for culture) would be indicated, to exclude infection of the ascitic fluid and peritonitis. The ascitic fluid can be tapped to dryness with IV albumin support (to prevent hypotension and shock).
Start frusemide and continue spironolactone.

Alcoholic liver disease is by far the commonest cause of liver failure. Women have an increased susceptibility to alcohol-induced liver damage. It is only in the presence of advanced alcoholic hepatitis or cirrhosis that the patient manifests clinical evidence of alcoholic liver disease. There are no definitive blood tests for this condition although, as in this case, the results of the full blood count, clotting studies and albumin may imply underlying chronic liver disease. The liver function tests may also be normal, even in the face of advanced liver damage. An EEG may confirm the onset of hepatic encephalopathy showing triphasic slow waves. Assessing arterial ammonia levels can be useful. A definitive diagnosis may be made at liver biopsy.

　Given this patient's clinical presentation, hepatic encephalopathy will obviously need to be excluded. In the absence of an infective cause (i.e. chest or urinary infection, infected ascitic fluid), treating the constipation and the electrolyte abnormalities will be the main focus of this patient's treatment. Ultimately, abstention from alcohol will be necessary, although established cirrhosis is irreversible. If abstention is successfully maintained, liver transplantation may be possible.

A 28-year-old Ugandan man was admitted to ITU. The history from his friends was that he had become increasingly unwell for a week, with shortness of breath and fever. He had taken to his bed and had stopped eating. Antibiotic treatment had already been initiated 48 hours earlier.

On examination, he was pyrexial at 38°C. There was cervical lymphadenopathy with bilateral coarse crepitations on auscultation.

The results of his investigations were as follows:
Hb 7.4 g/dl, Plts 215×10^9/l, WCC 6.5×10^9/l.
Blood film (day 2 of admission): fragmented red cells, reticulocytosis.
G6PD status: 0.7 IU/g haemoglobin (4.6–13.5).
Clotting and fibrinogen: normal.
Coombs' test: positive.

Sodium 127 mmol/l, potassium 3.8 mmol/l, urea 4.9 mmol/l creatinine 106 µmol/l.
Blood gases on air: Po_2 7.1 kPa, Pco_2 3.76 kPa, standard bicarbonate 21.6 mmol/l, B.E. −3.9.
Chest radiograph: widespread reticulo-nodular shadowing in both fields.

A Give the likely diagnosis.

B How would you explain the patient's blood film?

A *Mycoplasma pneumoniae.* ✱✱✱
Pneumocystis carinii pneumonia. ✱✱
Miliary tuberculosis. ✱✱

B Coombs' positive haemolysis secondary to mycoplasma pneumonia, with perhaps a contribution from haemolysis secondary to G6PD deficiency triggered by cotrimoxazole or septicaemia *per se*.

In this case a young Ugandan man presented with a short history of respiratory failure and evidence of haemolysis on blood film after initiation of antibiotic treatment. Given the patient's ethnic background, HIV seropositivity has to be considered, suggesting a possible diagnosis of *Pneumocystis carinii* pneumonia in this case. It is a reasonable assumption therefore that this man was treated with intravenous high-dose cotrimoxazole, which in the presence of his G6PD deficiency could lead to intravascular haemolysis. Septicaemia alone could also be a trigger for haemolysis in the latter condition. Other drugs which may trigger haemolysis in G6PD deficiency include dapsone, nitrofurantoin, primaquine, ciprofloxacin and other sulphonamide antibiotics.

However, this would not explain his Coombs' positive haemolysis. The Coombs' test, or positive direct antiglobulin test, detects antibody-covered red blood cells by their agglutination with antihuman antibody. It is divided into 'warm' and 'cold' types depending on whether binding of anti-red cell antibody occurs at or below body temperature. 'Warm' types are said to be due to IgG or complement covering the red cells, and this type of haemolysis can occur in, for example, systemic lupus erythematosus (SLE), chronic lymphocytic leukaemia or Hodgkin's disease. 'Cold' agglutinins are due to binding of IgM and are said to occur in (for example) lymphoma or macroglobulinaemia, and in infections such as mycoplasma, malaria and trypanosomiasis.

A diagnosis of mycoplasma would explain the respiratory failure along with the Coombs' positive haemolysis. Malaria obviously has to be ruled out as a cause of the latter, in a man who has lived predominantly in Uganda, but this alone would not explain the chest pathology.

Coombs' positive haemolysis is said to cause auto-agglutination, reticulocytosis and occasionally fragmentation of red cells on the blood film, especially if cold agglutinins, which cause intravascular haemolysis, are involved. Haemolysis in G6PD deficiency classically has a film showing irregular contracted cells, with bite cells and blister cells. Heinz bodies within the red cells are said to be characteristic.

Finally, tuberculosis should always be considered in an African patient presenting with respiratory failure. Although this usually presents more chronically, it can have a rapid presentation in the context of immunosuppression.

An 83-year-old man was seen as an out-patient, with a 5-month history of weight loss and malaise. Examination revealed stony dullness at the left base with a heart rate of 64/min and normal heart sounds. The patient was admitted for further evaluation. A pleural tap on admission yielded 300 ml of blood-stained fluid, with a protein content of 45 g/l, glucose of 3 mmol/l and negative Gram and Ziehl–Neelsen stains.

His other test results are shown below:
Hb 9.9 g/dl, MCV 85 fl, total WCC 5.0×10^9/l, Plts 141×10^9/l.
ESR 76 mm/h.

Sodium 142 mmol/l, potassium 5.4 mmol/l, bicarbonate 26 mmol/l, urea 18.8 mmol/l, creatinine 205 µmol/l, albumin 25 g/l, alkaline phosphatase 134 IU/l, bilirubin 8 µmol/l, ALT 17 IU/l, serum total protein 35 g/l, serum glucose 7 mmol/l, thyroxine 83 nmol/l.

Chest radiograph: pleural calcification visible along left diaphragmatic border (after pleural tap).

A What is the type of pleural effusion described above?
   Give the differential diagnosis of this type of pleural effusion.

B In view of the above results, what is the likeliest diagnosis and what tests would you perform to elucidate this further?

A Exudative pleural effusion. ✱✱✱

The differential diagnosis of an exudative pleural effusion depends on whether it is unilateral or bilateral. Causes of unilateral pleural effusion include malignancy (bronchial carcinoma, mesothelioma, lymphoma), infection (secondary to pneumonia, empyema or tuberculous) and infarction (secondary to a pulmonary embolus).

Causes of bilateral pleural effusion include malignancy (disseminated metastases), connective tissue disease, rheumatoid arthritis, vasculitides, asbestosis and post-pericardiotomy syndrome.

An exudative pleural effusion is characterized by a protein level of >30 g/l and an LDH level of >200 IU/l. Further characterization is provided by a glucose level relative to serum glucose, in that the former is reduced in infectious, malignant and rheumatoid effusions. Amylase level in an effusion is high in those secondary to pancreatitis or oesophageal perforation. Effusions may be chylous if there has been trauma to the thoracic duct or in the presence of lymphoma. pH is reduced in oesophageal rupture (<6.0) and to a lesser extent in empyema.

B Mesothelioma. ✱✱✱
Tuberculosis. ✱

The pleural tap gave a blood-stained exudate. Heavy blood-staining occurs in malignant involvement of the pleura, as a result of pulmonary infarction or in tuberculosis. Pleural calcification is found as a result of mesothelioma, asbestosis or tuberculous empyema. Given the history of weight loss and malaise, the differential is between malignant involvement of the pleura or tuberculosis (despite the lack of AAFB in the pleural aspirate). A CT of the chest and/or fine-needle aspiration biopsy would differentiate these , although needle biopsy with mesothelioma should be avoided, if possible, as the tumour may spread along the needle track.

A 36-year-old woman was seen in the casualty room with a 3-day history of numbness of the right hand, pain behind the right eye, diplopia on right lateral gaze, intermittent blurring of vision, increased weakness and clumsiness of the right hand and a one-day history of a headache and a stiff neck. She had never had symptoms like this in the past. She was 3 weeks post-partum after the birth of her first baby. The past medical history was normal apart from 'borderline' diabetes mellitus during her pregnancy.

Neurological examination showed altered sensation to light touch in the ophthalmic division of the trigeminal nerve. There was no clinical ophthalmoplegia but she complained of diplopia on looking to the right. The upper limbs showed normal tone and reflexes but the right arm was slightly weaker than the left in all muscle groups. Lower-limb tone and reflexes were again normal but the right leg was weaker than the left in all muscle groups. The plantar responses were flexor. The patient complained of pain on neck flexion but Kernig's sign was negative.

A What is the likeliest cause of this woman's problems?

B What tests would you request?

A Dissociative syndrome. ✱✱✱
   Demyelination. ✱✱

B MRI brain and cervical cord. ✱✱✱
   Lumbar puncture for oligoclonal bands. ✱✱
   Trimodal evoked potentials including visually evoked (VEP), brainstem auditory (BSAEP) and upper-
   and lower-limb somatosensory (SSEP) evoked potentials. ✱✱
   FBC including eosinophil count. ✱
   Fasting glucose. ✱
   ANA/rheumatoid factor/ANCA/ESR (possible vasculitis). ✱
   Porphobilinogen (possible acute intermittent porphyria). ✱

This patient has no 'hard' neurological signs. For example, although she has a partial right hemiparesis her right plantar is flexor, and although she complains of diplopia and blurred vision, her cranial nerve examination was unremarkable. To fit her neurological symptoms with a neuro-anatomical location, one must postulate multiple pathological events at multiple sites. This may include demyelination (e.g. secondary to the first episode of multiple sclerosis), vasculitis, or other infectious/inflammatory or malignant CSF conditions. However, there is little in the history to support an organic aetiology.

A 35-year-old window cleaner was seen in casualty following a fall from his ladder. He was drowsy on admission and his recollection of how he fell was scanty. There was no focal neurology and the remainder of the examination was also unremarkable. A skull X-ray confirmed a right temporal fracture and a CT scan of the head showed a small quantity of blood in the anterior interhemispheric fissure, which was thought to be secondary to trauma. The patient's conscious level returned to normal by the next day and he was allowed to return home. One month later he was brought in comatose, having been found at home by a friend. He died later that evening.

A What was the likely cause of this man's second presentation?

B What additional investigation would you have included in your initial assessment on his first presentation?

A Massive subarachnoid haemorrhage from probable anterior communicating artery aneurysm. ✱✱✱
Subarachnoid haemorrhage. ✱

B Four-vessel cerebral angiography. ✱✱✱
Magnetic resonance angiography. ✱✱

Subarachnoid haemorrhage often presents as collapse of unknown origin. The true cause of the collapse can be masked if additional trauma has occurred, as in this case. This man's fall was caused by a small subarachnoid bleed from an anterior communicating artery aneurysm: failure to detect this by carrying out an angiogram resulted in a massive bleed from the same aneurysm a month later. Trauma *per se* is more often associated with subdural or extra-dural haematoma.

The decision to use angiography vs. MRA is debatable. Angiography carries a 1–2% risk of serious morbidity, e.g. stroke, in those above 60 years. MRA is safe but may miss smaller aneurysms. If surgery is contemplated, formal angiography will have to be done in any case. In this case, an underlying aneurysm is very likely and surgery would be contemplated.

A 28-year-old man was started on phenytoin and dexamethasone for a glioma detected on a CT scan of the brain. Five days later the house-physician was called to see him on the ward with a fever and hypotension. On examination, there was a widespread exfoliative skin rash present over the trunk and extremities with a positive Nikolsky's sign. The remainder of the examination was unremarkable.

The investigations were as follows:
Hb 12.3 g/dl, WCC 8.0×10^9/l, Plts 350×10^9/l.

Sodium 134 mmol/l, potassium 4.6 mmol/l, urea 7.0 mmol/l, creatinine 95 µmol/l.
Liver function tests normal.
ESR 55 mm/h.

A What condition has this man developed?

B Give the likely underlying cause.

C Give two other conditions that may cause a positive Nikolsky's sign.

A Toxic epidermal necrolysis. ✳✳✳

B Phenytoin. ✳✳✳
Staphylococcal scalded skin syndrome. ✳✳

C Porphyria cutanea tarda.
Pemphigus vulgaris.

Nikolsky's sign refers to the complete separation of the stratum corneum from the underlying epidermis as a single sheet of skin. This occurs in toxic epidermal necrolysis, which may be drug induced (e.g. secondary to sulphonamides, barbiturates, phenolphthalein and phenytoin) or may be secondary to staphylococcal phage type 71.

A 23-year-old woman was seen by the duty casualty officer. She had recently been diagnosed as epileptic and had been started on phenytoin. She was worried by increasing tiredness, malaise, nausea and vomiting. Her ankles had a tendency to swell at the end of the day. She was also on a salbutamol inhaler for mild asthma and took the oral contraceptive pill (OCP). Physical examination revealed an obese but otherwise normal young woman.

The following tests were conducted:
Hb 11.3 g/dl, WCC 6.5 × 10⁹/l, MCV 98 fl, Plts 380 × 10⁹/l.

Sodium 132 mmol/l, potassium 4.2 mmol/l, urea 3.5 mmol/l, creatinine 70 μmol/l, albumin 38 g/l.

A What has caused her problems?

B What further tests would you consider?

A Phenytoin causing inactivation of oestrogen in oral contraceptive pill (OCP). ✶✶✶
Phenytoin toxicity causing fatigue and nausea. ✶

Recent introduction of phenytoin has caused induction of hepatic cytochrome P_{450} metabolizing enzymes. This has increased the metabolism of the OCP, thereby reducing its activity. Other agents that may do this include carbamazepine, phenobarbitone, rifampicin, spironolactone and griseofulvin.
    Phenytoin toxicity can present with nausea and vomiting but cerebellar signs are also often noted.

B Pregnancy test. ✶✶✶
Phenytoin level. ✶

A 23-year-old man with known acquired immunodeficiency syndrome (AIDS) was seen in the out-patient clinic with a thyroid swelling. Further examination revealed cervical lymphadenopathy and hepatosplenomegaly. Thyroid function tests were subsequently found to be normal and a technetium 99^m scan revealed a cold thyroid nodule.

A What is the likely cause of this man's thyroid swelling?

B What further tests would you carry out to confirm your clinical suspicion?

A Lymphoma secondary to AIDS. ✱✱✱
Malignant metastasis. ✱
Localized thyroiditis. ✱
Adenoma. ✱
Thyroid abscess. ✱

B Excision biopsy of cold nodule. ✱✱✱
Lymph node biopsy. ✱✱
Ultrasound of abdomen. ✱✱

A 40-year-old insulin-dependent diabetic woman was seen in casualty with acute abdominal pain 5 hours after a drinking binge. She had a past medical history of depression and alcoholism. There was no alteration in bowel habit.

Abdominal examination revealed a soft, tender abdomen. On neurological examination the patient had poor short-term memory, reduced concentration span and a stocking distribution of loss of sensation to light touch with preserved vibration and joint position sense. Plantars were extensor and ankle jerks were diminished but present.

The initial investigations were as follows:

Sodium 130 mmol/l, potassium 4.8 mmol/l, urea 3.2 mmol/l, creatinine 125 µmol/l, bicarbonate 20 mmol/l, glucose 20 mmol/l, bilirubin 20 µmol/l, AST 25 IU/l, ALT 27 IU/l, alkaline phosphatase 100 IU/l, albumin 30 g/dl.

A Give the two likeliest causes of this woman's abdominal pain.

B Give two possible causes of her peripheral neuropathy.

A Pancreatitis. ✱✱✱
Diabetes mellitus. ✱✱

B Alcohol neuropathy. ✱✱✱
Diabetic neuropathy. ✱✱✱
B_{12} deficiency. ✱✱
Folate deficiency. ✱✱

This question serves to highlight some of the medical causes of acute abdomen; others to remember include acute intermittent porphyria, familial Mediterranean fever and lead poisoning.

Neuropathy due to B_{12} or folate deficiency tends to involve the posterior columns with both vibration and joint position sense loss. Furthermore, subacute combined degeneration, which can occur in the context of either B_{12} or folate deficiency, often has accompanying upper motor neurone signs (extensor plantars) with depressed ankle jerks.

An 18-year-old woman presented to her GP with a 2-month history of severe headaches and blurred vision. She had recently been started on the OCP, and was also on treatment for severe acne vulgaris. On examination, she was found to be obese with facial acne. Neurological examination revealed bilateral papilloedema.

A What condition is she likely to be suffering from?

B How would you confirm your diagnosis?

C What risk factors does this patient have for developing this condition?

D How would you treat this patient?

A Benign intracranial hypertension (BIH). ✱✱✱
Cerebral venous sinus occlusion causing raised intracranial pressure. ✱✱
Space-occupying lesion. ✱

B MRI/MRV brain. ✱✱✱
Lumbar puncture measuring intracranial pressure. ✱✱
CT brain. ✱✱

C Tetracyclines/retinoids for treatment of acne vulgaris.
Obesity.
OCP.

D Stop all possible precipitating drugs.
Encourage weight loss.
Repeated lumbar punctures to remove cerebrospinal fluid.
Acetazolamide/frusemide.
Visual acuity check.
Baseline Goldmann perimetry to exclude peripheral visual field constriction.
Ventriculo-peritoneal shunt or consideration of optic nerve fenestration for resistant cases.

In any case of suspected BIH, an MRV needs to be carried out to exclude cerebral venous sinus thrombosis, which has increasingly been found to be an underlying cause in cases of BIH. If venous thrombosis is found, current management is intravenous heparin followed by warfarinization.

The intracranial pressure in BIH needs to be controlled as damage to peripheral visual fields and eventually drop in visual acuity can occur. The baseline visual field should be assessed by Goldmann perimetry and if this is abnormal, success of treatment can be monitored by subsequent improvement in visual fields.

Medically resistant cases or those with early visual field/acuity involvement may need surgical therapy with ventriculo-peritoneal shunting or optic nerve fenestration to relieve pressure on the optic nerve.

A 65-year-old vagrant was diagnosed as having pulmonary tuberculosis, following a bronchoscopy. He was started on the appropriate therapy but failed to attend several follow-up appointments. He eventually reappeared, 5 months after starting treatment, complaining of diarrhoea, poor sleep, a sore mouth and weight loss.

On examination, he had a scarlet, enlarged tongue and a brown scaly rash over his hands and around his neck and anterior chest wall. The following full blood count was obtained:
Hb 8.3 g/dl, MCV 104 fl, WCC 3.8×10^9/l, Plts 110×10^9/l.

A What eponymous term is given to the rash around this patient's neck?

B What is the cause of his presenting symptoms?

C Give a possible risk factor that has led to this condition.

D Give a cause of his macrocytosis.

E What might iron staining of his bone marrow illustrate?

A Casal's necklace.

B Pellagra.

C Alcoholism. ✳✳✳
Isoniazid toxicity. ✳✳
Poor compliance with taking pyridoxine supplement. ✳✳

D Alcohol. ✳✳✳
Liver dysfunction secondary to alcohol or antituberculous drugs. ✳✳✳
Sideroblastic anaemia secondary to alcohol or isoniazid. ✳✳
Co-existing folate deficiency due to poor diet. ✳✳
Dietary B_{12} deficiency. ✳✳

E Ring sideroblasts in the bone marrow.

The classic triad for pellagra is diarrhoea, dermatitis and dementia. The presentation may be less clear cut, with poor sleep, lack of concentration, confusion and weight loss. The classical rash develops on sun-exposed areas of skin and is initially erythematous, giving way to scaly, brown discoloration. The antituberculous drug isoniazid is usually given with pyridoxine (vitamin B_6). In excess, it will prevent pyridoxine activation. This in turn depletes niacin (vitamin B_3), resulting in pellagra.

A 72-year-old woman was admitted to hospital, having collapsed at home. She had been found by her close friend who cared for her and who gave the majority of the history. Two months previously, the woman had developed a rash on her chest and legs, followed by bruising. She had subsequently suffered from shortness of breath on exertion, weakness and falls. She had been seen by her GP, who prescribed a course of antibiotics. Her past medical history included rheumatoid arthritis, for which she was under specialist care. She was on two sets of pills, but couldn't remember their names.

On examination, she was pale and pyrexial. She had cervical lymphadenopathy and a petechial rash present over her chest and legs, with bruising over her bottom. She was tachycardic with a blood pressure of 120/60 mmHg. She had bronchial breathing at the left base on auscultation, and abdominal examination revealed a three-finger breadth liver and four-finger breadth splenic enlargement.

The following investigations were performed:

Sodium 136 mmol/l, potassium 4.1 mmol/l, urea 5.9 mmol/l, creatinine 96 µmol/l, glucose 11.8 mmol/l, bicarbonate 23 mmol/l, calcium 2.26 mmol/l, phosphate 0.94 mmol/l, bilirubin 18 µmol/l, albumin 33 g/l, ALT 18 IU/l, alkaline phosphatase 51 mmol/l.
Hb 4.6 g/dl, WCC 85×10^9/l, Plts 30×10^9/l.
PT 22 s, APTT 42 s, fibrinogen 0.8 g/l.

Chest radiograph: absent stomach bubble; raised left hemi-diaphragm; diffuse shadowing left lung base.

A   What is the likely cause of this patient's acute presentation?

B   What is the likely underlying diagnosis?

C   How would you confirm this diagnosis?

D   What clotting abnormality does she manifest?

E   What would be your acute management of this case?

F   What is the danger of giving a blood transfusion to this patient?

A Pneumonia secondary to relative immunosuppression. ✳✳✳
Tuberculosis. ✳

B Acute promyelocytic leukaemia (M3). ✳✳✳
Acute myelocytic leukaemia. ✳✳

C Blood film looking for blast cells.
Bone marrow: may show typical hypergranular blasts with cytoplasmic, azurophilic Auer rods (virtually pathognomonic of AML).

D Disseminated intravascular coagulation (DIC).

E Rehydration and oxygen.
Broad-spectrum antibiotics: piperacillin and gentamicin.
Careful blood transfusion to <10 g/dl.
Platelet transfusion.
Fresh frozen plasma (FFP) infusion.
Prophylactic heparin is advised by some for type M3 AML.

F In view of the very high white cell count, blood transfusion to >10 g/dl may increase whole blood viscosity appreciably, leading to leucostasis and the movement of leucocyte thrombi to the brain, lungs and heart.

The presentation of the above patient with a chest infection, elevated white cell count and DIC is typical of the M3 variant of AML. After acute supportive treatment, remission induction chemotherapy with daunorubicin, Ara-C (cytosine arabinoside) and 6 thioguanine (DAT) would be considered.

A 70-year-old man was seen in the out-patient clinic complaining of weakness in his arms and legs and the sensation of his muscles 'jumping'. His problems had started 6 months earlier, with sudden-onset weakness of his left hand over the course of a week. He had been seen by his GP who had prescribed aspirin. Despite this treatment the weakness had spread to his left arm and leg. Three weeks prior to admission, he had noticed weakness of his right hand. He had become increasingly unsteady and was prone to falls. He had also become aware of his speech slurring and his muscles twitching. He was a smoker with occasional alcohol use, and he had noticed a loss in weight of one stone over the 6 months prior to admission.

On examination, the patient was emaciated. Cardiorespiratory and abdominal examination was normal. Cranial nerve examination was unremarkable with a normal jaw jerk and no tongue fasciculation. Examination of the upper limbs revealed generalized fasciculation over the biceps and triceps of both arms and also over the back. There was wasting of the small muscles of the hands bilaterally. The power of the right arm was reduced in all muscle groups to grade 4–/5. Upper limb reflexes were brisk and sensation was normal. In the lower limb there was bilateral wasting of the quadriceps with occasional fasciculation over the right quadriceps muscle. The muscle tone was normal bilaterally. Muscle power was reduced to grade 4+/5 in a pyramidal distribution in both legs. The knee jerk reflexes were hyper-reflexic bilaterally with normal ankle jerks. The plantar responses were withdrawal. The soft-touch and pin-prick sensations were both reduced over the dorsum of the right foot and over the anterior part of the right shin. Sacral sensation was normal, as was anal tone.

A Give a differential diagnosis for fasciculation in a general setting.

B Give the likely diagnosis for this patient's problems.

C What structure is it important to image?

D What further investigations would you carry out to confirm the diagnosis?

A Motor neuronopathy, i.e. destruction of α motor neurones (seen in motor neurone disease, spinal muscular atrophy and poliomyelitis).
Severe axonal motor neuropathy.
Some myopathies, e.g. polymyositis and inclusion body myositis.

B Motor neurone disease. ✳✳✳
Cervical myelopathy with additional cervical root compression. ✳✳
Multi-focal motor neuropathy with conduction block (MMNCB). ✳
Kennedy's disease (X-linked bulbospinal atrophy). ✳

C Cervical spine.

D Nerve conduction studies (NCS)/EMG. ✳✳✳
CT/MRI brain. ✳✳
Lumbar puncture: protein may be raised in MMNCB. ✳
Anti-ganglioside antibodies may be indicative of MMNCB. ✳

This elderly man has weight loss, lower motor neurone signs and soft upper motor neurone signs in the limbs. There are no signs above the foramen magnum and therefore it is especially important to exclude significant cervical cord and root compression. The lack of hard upper motor neurone signs in the presence of normal cord imaging would necessitate exclusion of MMNCB. This latter condition is thought of as a motor variant of chronic inflammatory demyelinating polyneuropathy (CIDP), and detailed NCS with proximal sampling should be carried out to exclude significant motor conduction block due to regional demyelination. The condition is eminently treatable with intravenous immunoglobulin. Kennedy's disease is a trinucleotide repeat disorder with CAG repeats within the androgen gene on the X chromosome. As with MMNCB it gives purely lower motor neurone signs and an additional sensory neuropathy may be present. Bulbar signs —which this man does not manifest— are usually prominent . A genetic test is available to screen for this rare disorder. Contrary to common teaching, soft sensory signs may be permissible in motor neurone disease, especially in elderly patients.

The majority of patients in whom a diagnosis of motor neurone disease is entertained should have imaging of the brain and a lumbar puncture to rule out inflammatory/malignant CSF processes, which can rarely give a similar clinical phenotype. CSF protein may also be raised in MMNCB as with CIDP. Although NCS/EMG is helpful in establishing a diagnosis of motor neurone disease, the overall diagnosis is clinical.

A 23-year-old homosexual man was seen in casualty, complaining of weakness on his right-hand side. He had been treated for a *Pneumocystis carinii* pneumonia 2 months previously and it was shortly after this that he had noticed his right foot dragging on walking. Over the last month he had found it difficult to fasten his shirt buttons and ties. His performance at work had deteriorated and he had become increasingly forgetful with poor concentration.

On examination, he was emaciated and had facial *molluscum contagiosum*. Neurological examination revealed right hemiparesis. The cranial nerves were intact and his mental test score was 22/30.

The initial investigations were as follows:
Hb 10.5 g/dl, MCV 83 fl, WCC 2.5×10^9/l, Plts 250×10^9/l.
Sodium 132 mmol/l, potassium 4.2 mmol/l, urea 4.0 mmol/l, creatinine 68 µmol/l.
ESR 28 mm/h, CD_4 count: 50 cells/mm^3.

A What further investigations would you request?

B What is the likely cause of this man's neurological features?

C How would you treat him?

A HIV test. ✱✱✱
MRI brain (if not available then CT brain with contrast). ✱✱✱
Serum toxoplasma antigen. ✱✱

Lumbar puncture (if no space-occupying lesion on the brain scan) with PCR for JC virus, cell count, protein, glucose, India ink stain (to identify *Cryptococcus neoformans*), Ziehl–Neelsen staining; TB PCR, cytospin and clonal typing of cells. ✱✱

B Progressive myeloid leucoencephalopathy (PML). ✱✱✱
Cerebral toxoplasmosis. ✱✱
Cerebral lymphoma. ✱✱
Cerebral cryptococcomata. ✱
AIDS–dementia complex. ✱
Infective cerebral abscess. ✱

C Normal practice in this case is to treat for toxoplasmosis with sulphadiazine and pyrimethamine and look for a clinical response with a change in appearance of the lesions on re-scanning. If there is no response to treatment it is worth considering stereotactic biopsy of the lesion, as pyogenic infective abscess is a possibility, although there is little in the history to suggest an active infection. AIDS–dementia complex has both behavioural and motor signs but these are rarely manifest as a focal neurological lesion. PML may show some response to zidofovir.

The likeliest diagnosis in this particular case lies between PML, cerebral toxoplasmosis and cerebral lymphoma. All three can be of insidious onset with focal neurological features; one should be able to differentiate between them on imaging as PML presents as high-signal demyelinating white matter lesions on MRI. If ring-enhancing lesions are seen on the brain scan the differential lies between cerebral toxoplasmosis and lymphoma. Lymphoma may also show a periventricular predilection.

A 49-year-old epileptic man was seen in casualty. He had recently been noted to be confused, with difficulty in walking. There had been a change in his speech. He had recently been seen by his GP for epigastric pain that was diagnosed as indigestion.

On examination, he had coarse features, gingival hyperplasia and was drowsy. He had a normal Glasgow Coma Scale score. On neurological examination, he had nystagmus, finger–nose ataxia and a slurring dysarthria.

The initial investigations were as follows:
Hb 9.8 g/dl, MCV 105 fl, WCC 5.5×10^9/l, Plts 190×10^9/l.
Urea and electrolytes normal.

A What is the underlying cause of this man's deterioration?

B What is the likely cause of his haematological abnormality and how would you treat it?

A Phenytoin toxicity secondary to inhibition of metabolism caused by cimetidine. ✱✱✱
Phenytoin toxicity. ✱✱

B The patient is also folate deficient, which can occur in at-risk groups such as the elderly, those with poor nutrition, alcoholics and patients on chronic anticonvulsant therapy. He should be started on folate replacement therapy.

This man was prescribed cimetidine by his GP for his indigestion. Some antibiotics (e.g. erythromycin and metronidazole) and other drugs (e.g. chlorpromazine, allopurinol and cimetidine) cause inhibition of hepatic cytochrome P_{450}. This in turn elevates the serum phenytoin level. Phenytoin toxicity may result, producing drowsiness and cerebellar signs, as in this case.

A 20-year-old woman presented acutely with collapse and reduced GCS. She required intubation as she was not protecting her airway. Her family gave a 3-month history of unsteady gait and slurring of speech. Three years earlier she had suffered a retinal detachment in her left eye secondary to haemorrhage from a retinal haemangioma. The eye had to be enucleated because of chronic pain. A year later, she suffered a detached retina in the right eye. Her father had died of a renal cell carcinoma in his early forties. Her brother, paternal aunt and paternal cousin had all had similar eye problems. On clinical evaluation, she had papilloedema with intact corneal and doll's eye reflexes. She was intubated and ventilated. She had limb withdrawal to painful stimuli with brisk reflexes, bilateral sustained ankle clonus and extensor plantars.

A What is the cause of her current presentation?

B What is the underlying condition?

C What investigations would you request?

A Acute bleed from cerebellar haemangioblastoma. **✳✳✳**
Acute bleed from cerebellar arterio-venous malformation. **✳✳**
Bleed into cerebellar mass lesion. **✳**

B Von Hippel–Lindau (VHL) syndrome.

C CT brain to establish bleed into posterior fossa. **✳✳✳**
MRI/MRA brain. **✳✳**
Formal four-vessel angiography as prelude to neurosurgery. **✳✳**
Genetic testing for VHL locus on 3p25–26. **✳✳**
Elective CT scan of abdomen to exclude renal, hepatic and pancreatic lesions. **✳**

Von Hippel–Lindau syndrome results in retinal and cerebellar haemangioblastomata, renal and pancreatic cysts, renal cell carcinoma, phaeochromocytoma and less frequently haemangioblastomata in other sites, such as spinal cord and medulla. The earliest lesion is often a retinal haemangioblastoma, which may bleed and lead to retinal detachment and secondary glaucoma. Cerebellar haemangioblastomata are found in up to 60% of cases and can present chronically with ataxia, dysarthria, nystagmus and headache or more rarely with an acute bleed. Bleeds into the posterior fossa are of particular concern due to blockage of the fourth ventricle and subsequent raised intracranial pressure and coning.

Hypernephromata are identified in 45% of affected individuals at autopsy and present in the early forties. Screening of affected individuals for retinal tumours should begin in childhood; it should continue throughout life with CT brain, ultrasound scans of the kidneys and urinary catecholamines being conducted annually.

A 17-year-old boy was referred to the neurology out-patient clinic complaining of painful cramps after exercise. His problems had started at the age of 14 when he became aware of cramps following sport at school. These would last for up to 10 minutes. Between the ages of 14 and 17 the frequency of these attacks became worse, but he had no overt weakness and could keep up with the other boys. In the month prior to being seen, he had developed pain in the inner aspect of his thighs, which was sharp and fleeting in nature. The cramps affected his arms and his legs and he had one attack in bed. There was no history of pigmenturia, rashes, arthropathy, steroid usage or second wind phenomenon. He was treated with quinine by his GP with little response.

On examination, he was short for his age. There was no rash present. Cardiological examination revealed a soft ejection systolic murmur over the fourth intercostal space with no radiation to the carotid arteries or aortic area. Neurological examination was essentially normal apart from slight weakness of hip flexion, graded 4+/5. All reflexes were normal.

The initial investigations showed a normal full blood count, urea and electrolytes, lactate and pyruvate. The CPK was 900 IU/l.

A What is the diagnosis?

B How would you confirm your diagnosis?

A McArdle's syndrome. ✶✶✶
Idiopathic cramps. ✶

B Muscle biopsy.

The history above is typical for McArdle's syndrome. This is classified as a type V glycogen storage disorder. The disease may present in childhood with fatigue, leading to muscular cramps on exertion in adult life, which may be accompanied by myoglobinuria. Proximal muscle weakness may develop and overt muscle wasting may become apparent in later life. The lifespan is normal, unlike some of the other related glycogen storage disorders, and there is no hypoglycaemia as in von Gierke's or Forbes' disease (types I and III, respectively). Exertion, in this disorder, may lead to increased levels of lactate dehydrogenase, CPK and aldolase. Diagnosis is on muscle biopsy, which shows typical central migration of muscle nuclei and subsarcolemmal glycogen deposition.

A 48-year-old man with AIDS presented with increasing difficulty in walking. He found that over the month prior to being seen, his legs had become increasingly stiff and he tended to catch his feet on paving stones. His CD_4 count was $10\,mm^{-3}$, and his previous AIDS-defining illnesses were oesophageal candidiasis, gastric Kaposi's sarcoma and cytomegalovirus (CMV) encephalitis. He was on acyclovir, fluconazole, AZT and DDI.

On examination, he had oral candidiasis, palatal Kaposi's sarcoma and seborrhoeic dermatitis. Neurologically, cranial nerve and upper limb examinations were unremarkable. In the lower limb, the patient had a spastic paraparesis with pyramidal weakness, pathologically brisk reflexes and extensor plantar responses. Joint position and vibration sensation were abnormal to the hips bilaterally, but soft touch and pain were normal and there was no sensory level. The CT brain scan was normal.

A What is the diagnosis?

B What investigations would you carry out?

A Vacuolar myelopathy. ✳✳✳
Spinal lymphoma. ✳✳
Toxoplasmosis. ✳
Kaposi's sarcoma. ✳
CMV/HSV/cryptococcal CSF infection. ✳
HIV leucoencephalopathy. ✳
Spinal infarction, e.g. from HIV idiopathic thrombocytopaenic purpura (ITP) or HIV-associated arteritis. ✳

B MRI brain, cervical and thoracic cord. ✳✳✳
Lumbar puncture. ✳✳

The differential diagnosis of spastic paraparesis in the presence of HIV is wide. The above history would be typical for vacuolar myelopathy, which is found in up to 50% of AIDS patients at post-mortem. This is relatively insidious, with painless onset, ataxic paraparesis and sphincter disturbance with no sensory level. Vacuolation and monocytic infiltration of the long tracts and cord is found: the cause is unknown but direct infection by HIV is postulated.

A mass lesion compressing the cord is less likely in the above scenario in the absence of a sensory level. Lymphoma may be of B-cell origin or metastasis from a non-Hodgkin's lymphoma.

A 49-year-old woman was admitted as an emergency, with a sudden onset of aphasia on the day of admission. She had experienced a transient episode of right-sided weakness the previous week. She had had a mitral valve replacement 10 years previously and was taking sotalol, frusemide/amiloride combination diuretic and warfarin. She had recently been commenced on carbamazepine for trigeminal neuralgia. On examination, the patient was afebrile, her pulse being regular and blood pressure 140/90 mmHg. Cardiac auscultation revealed normal prosthetic valve sounds, with an ejection systolic murmur audible at the left sternal edge. She had an expressive and receptive dysphasia and a right upper motor neurone VII nerve palsy.

A Which investigations would you request?

B What is the most likely cause of this woman's symptoms?

A INR. ✳✳✳
CT scan of the brain. ✳✳✳
Transoesophageal echocardiogram. ✳

B Left middle cerebral artery (MCA) territory ischaemic infarct. ✳✳✳
Left MCA territory haemorraghic infarct. ✳✳
Transient ischaemic attack. ✳

This woman had sustained a left hemispheric ischaemic infarction in the MCA territory due to the action of carbamazepine in reducing the anticoagulant effect of warfarin. The main potential source of the cerebral embolus is likely to be from the mechanical mitral valve prosthesis. All patients with mechanical prosthetic heart valves will require lifelong anticoagulation. Patients with porcine heterografts are also anticoagulated for the first 3 months following valve insertion. Thereafter, its continuation depends on the position of the prosthesis (mitral prostheses being more thrombogenic than aortic prostheses, for instance) and the existence of other risk factors for thrombo-embolism such as atrial fibrillation.

An 18-year-old woman presented with an ileo-femoral venous thrombosis and pulmonary embolism. She was a smoker. There were no abnormal findings on examination. Since she was taking the OCP, this was withdrawn. She was anticoagulated with warfarin for 6 months. However, she was subsequently admitted with a further deep venous thrombosis and pulmonary embolism and was treated as previously, only for this to be followed by an episode of transient left hemiparesis. She was admitted for investigation.

A What are the possible diagnoses?

B What investigations would you request?

A Anti-phospholipid syndrome. ✳✳✳✳
Activated protein C resistance (Factor V Leiden). ✳✳✳
Congenital deficiencies of antithrombin III, protein S or C or factor II 20210 A mutation. ✳✳
SLE. ✳

B Clotting studies: including prothrombin time, KCCT, thrombin time, fibrinogen, antithrombin III, protein S and C levels, test for activated protein C resistance (Factor V Leiden), lupus anticoagulant. ✳✳✳
Anti-phospholipid antibody titres: Ig G and Ig M. ✳✳✳
Syphilis serology. ✳✳✳
dsDNA antibody titre and antinuclear factor. ✳✳
CT brain. ✳

An increased thromboembolic risk was present in this woman. She had no clinical features of SLE, in which there can be a history of thromboses, neurological disorder, thrombocytopenia and recurrent foetal loss. This may be associated with the lupus anticoagulant and anti-phospholipid antibodies. In the absence of clinical SLE and dsDNA antibodies, the diagnosis is more likely to be anti-phospholipid syndrome.

A congenital predisposition to thrombosis is rare. It should be considered in patients with an unexplained thrombotic episode who are below 40 years, have had recurrent deep venous thromboses or pulmonary embolism and have a positive family history for thromboembolic disease. Activated protein C resistance is the commonest of the congenital group of disorders. Protein C is a vitamin K-dependent protein that inhibits coagulation. Activated protein C acts by proteolytic cleavage of factors Va and VIIIa (both procoagulant proteins). Protein C resistance may result from a mutation in the activated protein C cleavage site of factor V (factor V Leiden), resulting in thrombophilia to a lesser (heterozygotes) or greater (homozygotes) degree.

The commonest form of homocystinuria, cystathionine β-synthase deficiency, may present as recurrent arterial occlusion (including renal, cerebral or coronary arteries). The morbidity and mortality is high below the age of 30. In this case, however, arterial and venous thromboses are seen. In addition, other clinical features of homocystinuria are absent — for example, lens dislocation and osteoporosis.

A 22-year-old woman was seen in casualty having returned from a 10-week trip to Thailand that morning. She had a 5-day history of fever, rigors and a dry cough. She had a severe headache and malaise but no photophobia or neck stiffness. She had been immunized against polio, tetanus, typhoid, and hepatitis A and B before departure but had taken no regular malaria prophylaxis. She had been trekking at high altitude and recalled receiving many insect bites.

On examination, her face, thorax and abdomen were markedly erythematous. The erythematous rash blanched easily on gentle pressure. She had tender cervical and inguinal lymphadenopathy. She had a heart rate of 120/min with a blood pressure of 110/70 mmHg. An abdominal examination revealed right inguinal discomfort. A vaginal examination revealed right adnexal tenderness and cervical excitation, with copious off-white vaginal discharge.

The following investigations were performed:
Hb 12.5 g/dl, total WCC 3.0×10^9/l, Plts 95×10^9/l, neutrophils 56.2%, lymphocytes 32%, monocytes 9.3%, eosinophils 0.4%, basophils 2.1%.
Blood film: no malarial parasites; reactive lymphocytes seen.
PT 17 s, APTT 50 s, fibrinogen 2.1 g/l.

Sodium 127 mmol/l, potassium 3.4 mmol/l, bicarbonate 25 mmol/l, urea 3.2 mmol/l, creatinine 79 μmol/l, glucose 5.2 mmol/l, albumin 36 g/l, alkaline phosphatase 44 IU/l, ALT 146 IU/l, bilirubin 8 μmol/l.

A What is the likely diagnosis?

B How would you manage this patient?

A Dengue fever. *******
Malaria. ******
Gonococcal septicaemia. ******
Co-existing pelvic inflammatory disease. *****
Lyme disease. *****

The clues to dengue fever in the above question include the reference to hilly areas of Thailand where dengue is often endemic (and where the ambient temperature is too cold to support the malarial parasite). The presentation with severe headache, prostration, an erythematous rash, tender lymphadenopathy and disseminated intravascular coagulation (DIC) is also supportive of this. The course of the illness is 7–10 days and may result in either complete recovery or shock with encephalitis, intracranial haemorrhage and liver failure.

The investigations in dengue fever often show a relative lymphopenia (with atypical lymphocytes on the blood film), thrombocytopenia, clotting abnormalities, hyponatraemia and a raised alanine transaminase.

Dengue fever is part of a family of viral haemorrhagic fevers, which include other flaviviruses such as yellow fever, arena viruses (e.g. Lassa fever), bunyaviruses (e.g. Congo–Crimean fever) and nosocomially spread filoviruses (e.g. Marburg and Ebola).

Of the other possibilities, both malaria and gonococcal disease can cause DIC. However, as already pointed out, malaria is rarely found in high altitude areas and although a normal white cell count is not unusual in gonococcal disease, one would not expect reactive lymphocytes on the blood film, which are more suggestive of a viral aetiology. Although Lyme disease is also endemic in these areas of Thailand, and the history of multiple insect bites acquired during trekking is suggestive, the rash and clinical picture is quite different.

B The treatment of dengue fever is entirely symptomatic and involves treatment of shock with inotropic support if necessary, and adequate replacement of blood products to compensate for the DIC.

A 55-year-old woman was seen in the out-patient clinic complaining of deafness and tinnitus affecting her left ear. Her problems had started 2 months earlier following a bout of coryza. Her GP had prescribed a course of antibiotics following a physical examination. She had also recently had the sensation of the room spinning around her.

Physical examination revealed normal tympanic membranes bilaterally. The corneal reflex was absent on the left and she had a lower motor neurone VII palsy on the same side. She was Rinne positive on both sides and Weber's test was referred to her right hand side.

The results of the investigations were as follows:
Hb 12.5 g/dl, WCC 5.5×10^9/l, Plts 190×10^9/l.
ESR 40 mm/h.
Urea and electrolytes normal.

A What is the likely underlying diagnosis?

B What is the investigation of choice?

A Left acoustic neuroma. ✱✱✱
Left acoustic schwannoma. ✱✱✱
Left cerebellopontine angle glioma. ✱✱
Left cerebellopontine angle meningioma. ✱✱

B Magnetic resonance scan of cerebellopontine angle. This is the investigation of choice for lesions in the posterior fossa.

This is a classical presentation for an acoustic neuroma. The corneal reflex is often lost early on, due to compression of the fibres of Va at the cerebellopontine angle. Hemi-anaesthesia, hemiparesis, limb ataxia and cranial nerve palsies affecting VI, VII and VIII may also occur. Bilateral acoustic neuromas are found in neurofibromatosis type 2 (gene on long arm chromosome 22).

A 60-year-old woman presented with a 3-week history of malaise, dyspnoea and pleuritic chest pain. She had a history of carcinoma of the breast 20 years previously, which required mastectomy. On examination, she was febrile, pulse 110 min^{-1} regular with chest signs consistent with a left pleural effusion. She had marked left-sided chest wall tenderness.

Her initial investigations were as follows:
Hb 10.2 g/dl, WCC 23.1 × 10^9/l (neutrophils 90%), platelets 580 × 10^9/l.
Arterial blood gases on air: pH 7.45, P_{CO_2} 4.2 kPa, P_{O_2} 9.8 kPa.
Chest radiograph: left lower and mid-zone shadowing with an air bronchogram present.
Left-sided pleural effusion noted.

In spite of treatment with clarithromycin, clinical improvement failed to occur. She remained febrile and unwell with a persistent leucocytosis. The antibiotic therapy was reviewed and she was commenced on cefotaxime in addition to her previous therapy. Four days later, she remained febrile, with a WCC of 19.9 × 10^9/l.

A What is the most likely diagnosis?

B What further investigation would aid in making the diagnosis?

C What are the possible complications?

A Empyema. ✱✱✱
Lung abscess. ✱✱
Tuberculosis. ✱✱
Pulmonary metastases. ✱

B Pleural aspiration (with samples of the aspirate sent for microscopy, culture, sensitivities and cytology). ✱✱✱
CT scan of the thorax. ✱✱

C Discharge of the empyema through the chest wall (empyema necessitatis), into a bronchus (bronchopleural fistula) or spread to involve the pericardium (pericardial empyema). Even after healing, residual fibrosis and calcification may cause restriction of the underlying lung.

An empyema may be present even in the absence of a recent history of chest infection. The failure of this patient to improve clinically, a persistent temperature and polymorphonuclear leucocytosis all suggest that an empyema is the underlying problem. This may be confirmed by performing a pleural aspiration, when purulent fluid is aspirated. Drainage of the empyema often necessitates the insertion of an intercostal drain. A lung abscess, tuberculosis and pulmonary metastases (from the patient's previous breast carcinoma) will need to be considered in the differential diagnosis of her chest signs.

A 60-year-old man was referred to the medical out-patients' department with a history of malaise, weight loss, vague colicky abdominal pain, nausea and vomiting. On examination, he was seen to be pale and to have generalized abdominal tenderness, particularly in the left upper quadrant, with palpable splenomegaly. There were yellowish-brown skin plaques, which had a tendency to urticate and were pruritic on rubbing. There was no lymphadenopathy.

His initial investigations were as follows:
Hb 12.4 g/dl, Plts 181 × 10^9/l, WCC 6.8 × 10^9/l: neutrophils 3.2 × 10^9/l (48%), lymphocytes 1.97 × 10^9/l (30%), monocytes 1.22 × 10^9/l (15%), eosinophils 0.41 × 10^9/l (7%).
Plasma viscosity 1.88.
Liver function tests normal.

A What is the likely diagnosis?

B What tests would you perform to aid in diagnosis?

A Systemic mastocytosis. ✱✱✱
Acute monocytic leukaemia (AML). ✱✱
Chronic myelomonocytic leukaemia (CMML). ✱✱

B Bone marrow trephine and aspiration. ✱✱✱
CT abdomen. ✱

This man presents with malaise and non-specific symptoms. The differential diagnosis has to account for his monocytosis and splenomegaly. AML, CMML and systemic mastocytosis may all present with splenomegaly. In AML and CMML, lymphadenopathy is common, whilst in systemic mastocytosis it is not always present. Although systemic mastocytosis classically presents with skin lesions, particularly in children (urticaria pigmentosa), this is not essential. The skin lesions are characterized by their tendency to produce a wheal on rubbing due to the release of histamine from the mast cells (Darier's sign). A monocytosis may also occur in this condition. Bone marrow biopsy shows large numbers of mast cells, with normal lymphoid morphology, whilst in AML and CMML, blasts are present in significant numbers (>50% and <30%, respectively).

The medical registrar on call was asked to review a patient on the psychiatric ward. He was admitted with a psychotic episode and had been commenced on thioridazine. Although showing some initial improvement, he had subsequently become less mobile and had been noted to be pyrexial 2 days previously. On examination, he was orientated, had a regular tachycardia 110 min^{-1} with normal cardiac and chest auscultation. Neurological examination revealed generally increased limb tone but normal power and reflexes.

His investigations were as follows:
Hb 13 g/dl, WCC 9.1 × 10^9/l, Plts 300 × 10^9/l.
ECG: sinus tachycardia, no other abnormalities.

A What is the most likely diagnosis?

B What further tests may assist in confirming the diagnosis?

C How would you manage this patient?

A Neuroleptic malignant syndrome. ✱✱✱
Infection. ✱

B Creatinine phosphokinase (levels elevated during the illness). ✱✱✱
Blood cultures. ✱✱
Chest radiograph. ✱
Mid-stream urine. ✱

C Discontinue the thioridazine, with subsequent recovery taking up to 3 days following this. Dantrolene, levodopa and dopamine agonists all have been tried with some success.

The neuroleptic malignant syndrome is the idiosyncratic reaction to a phenothiazine, butyrophenone or thioxanthine resulting in a patient who is semiconscious, tachycardic, hyperthermic and has generally increased muscle tone. It usually develops over 1–3 days following the commencement of therapy and may take equally long to recover following withdrawal of the offending drug. A very similar syndrome is seen in parkinsonian patients on sudden withdrawal of dopamine agonists or levodopa. This procedure was previously done electively as a levodopa 'drug holiday' to treat dyskinesia. The fatalities that resulted from 'drug holidays' have led to a cessation of this treatment paradigm. Parkinsonian patients with this type of presentation have benefited from intravenous apomorphine (a dopamine agonist).

A 48-year-old tramp, well known to the casualty department, was brought into hospital after having collapsed in the street. He had a superficial graze to his left temple and smelt of alcohol. He was drowsy with a GCS of 10.

On examination, he was clubbed with palmar erythema, was jaundiced and had marked spider naevi on his upper torso. Abdominal examination revealed a distended abdomen with ascites, sparse secondary sexual hair and small genitalia. There was no organomegaly. Neurologically, he had a bilateral VI nerve palsy with both horizontal and vertical nystagmus. Pupils were meiotic and unreactive to both light and accommodation. Doll's eye reflexes were absent but the gag reflex was present. Limb examination revealed normal power and tone, but brisk reflexes with bilateral withdrawal on eliciting the plantar response.

The initial investigations were as follows:

Sodium 128 mmol/l, potassium 3.5 mmol/l, urea 1.2 mmol/l, creatinine 110 µmol/l, bicarbonate 22 mmol/l, glucose 2.0 mmol/l, albumin 25 g/l, ALT 35 IU/l, bilirubin 40 µmol/l, alkaline phosphatase 150 IU/l.
Hb 9.8 g/dl, MCV 102 fl, WCC 9.8×10^9/l, Plts 90×10^9/l.
PT 20 s.

A Give the likeliest cause of his neurological features.

B What further investigations would you request?

C What immediate treatment would you initiate?

A Wernicke's encephalopathy. ***
Central pontine myelinolysis. **
Brainstem intracerebral bleed. *
Hypoglycaemic coma. *

B MRI brain. ***
CT brain. *
Red cell transketolase. *
Lumbar puncture. *

C Give intravenous thiamine replacement followed by intravenous glucose in Casualty. It is dangerous to give glucose before thiamine. Thiamine pyrophosphate is the prosthetic group for transketolase and the substrate thiamine will be utilized in critically thiamine deficient patients. They will lose the small amount of this substrate remaining in the central nervous system as flux through the hexosemonophosphate shunt increases, risking acute Wernicke's encephalopathy which ultimately results in coma.

Initiate conservative treatment for hepatic encephalopathy with bowel clearance, vitamin K and multivitamin replacement and spironolactone.

This alcoholic patient presents with a combination of gaze paresis, depressed conscious level and possible long tract signs. This places any possible lesion within the mid-brain ± brain-stem. Central pontine myelinolysis can present with a very similar phenotype to Wernicke's and both can occur in alcoholics.

Typical signs seen in Wernicke's encephalopathy include an ocular palsy or other eye signs such as nystagmus, meiotic unreactive pupils or papilloedema; ataxia; confusion, apathy, stupor or coma. Diagnosis is essentially clinical although red cell transketolase activity can be useful if available. Treatment involves replacement of thiamine.

The medical registrar was asked to review a 65-year-old woman on the orthopaedic ward. She had undergone a knee replacement one week previously and was anticoagulated with warfarin, this being the routine practice. Three days later, with an INR of 2.5, she had a large haematemesis and passed 2 l of melaena per rectum. She denied any dyspepsia, before or subsequent to her admission. Her past medical history included an aortic graft, below the level of the renal arteries, 3 years previously. On examination, her pulse was 110 min^{-1}, BP 100/60, with some peri-umbilical pain and tenderness but no guarding, and bowel sounds were present.

Initial investigations were as follows:
Hb 8.2 g/dl, WCC 12 × 10^9/l, Plts 300 × 10^9/l, MCV 93 fl, MCH 29 pg.
Urea 10.2 mmol/l, creatinine 90 µmol/l.

Oesophagogastroduodenoscopy: some blood seen in the stomach; however, no bleeding point found in the upper gastrointestinal tract.

A Give two likely causes of this woman's blood loss.

B What further tests would you organize to establish the diagnosis?

A Paraprosthetic-enteric fistula. **✳✳**
Haemorrhage from a duodenal ulcer. **✳**

B Selective angiography (coeliac and superior mesenteric arteries). **✳✳✳**

In a patient of this age, bleeding from an upper gastrointestinal source is the likeliest cause of melaena, especially in the context of arthritis and probable use of non-steroidal anti-inflammatory drugs. Bleeding from such a source is not always visible at endoscopy.

In the presence of a large aortic aneurysm, a spontaneous fistula may rarely form to the duodenum. In the presence of an aortic graft, a paraprosthetic-enteric fistula may arise. If actively bleeding, this can be visualized by angiography, but otherwise may be difficult to detect. Endoscopy allows the distal areas of the duodenum to be visualized, at which point the opening of the fistula may be seen. Treatment is surgical intervention and closure of the fistula.

A 26-year-old woman was admitted with generalized seizures starting that afternoon. She was a known epileptic, having had her first seizure 6 years earlier. There was a family history of epilepsy with her elder sister having been diagnosed with idiopathic generalized epilepsy at the age of 10.

The patient had previously been admitted to numerous hospitals with the same complaint, requiring frequent ITU admissions. There were no focal neurological signs and she was afebrile. Following admission, she had a succession of tonic–clonic fits, which proved unresponsive to rectal diazepam (2 × 10 mg). She continued to fit unremittingly and had an apnoeic attack, during which she did not appear cyanosed, but spontaneously started breathing once more. She was subsequently given intravenous phenytoin (1000 mg over 30 min) which did not terminate the seizures. She was given propofol anaesthesia and thus required intubation and ventilatory support. An EEG carried out 12 hours after initiation of anaesthesia showed burst-suppression only.

A day later an attempt was made to wean propofol anaesthesia at the request of the neurologist. On coming round from anaesthesia the patient began to fit once again. Neurological examination during the seizure was normal with flexor plantars.

A What is the likely diagnosis?

B What investigations would you request?

C How would you proceed with treatment?

A Status epilepticus. ✱✱✱
Non-epileptic seizures. ✱✱

B Electrolytes including magnesium and calcium. ✱✱✱
Glucose. ✱✱✱
CT brain. ✱✱✱
Chase all old medical records. ✱✱✱
Lumbar puncture. ✱✱

C Check baseline and post-ictal prolactin levels
Continue ictal monitoring: if there is no EEG change correlating with clinical seizure, then this is suggestive of non-epileptic seizures. If this is the case, wean from the anaesthetic agent and all anti-epileptic medication.
If EEG confirms epileptic activity, re-anaesthetize with propofol and consider thiopentone anaesthesia. Check phenytoin levels and adjust accordingly. Load with intravenous phenobarbitone.

This scenario of a patient with adult onset epilepsy, an elder sister who has the disease and a past history of frequent ITU admissions for status epilepticus is suggestive of non-epileptic seizures. This supposition is further strengthened by the normal neurological examination during a seizure. However, the history could still be consistent with drug resistant status epilepticus and the patient needs to be investigated accordingly, especially before old notes are available.

These patients present a particular diagnostic challenge and fall under the diagnostic rubric of dissociative disorder. Ideal future management would include video-telemetry with concurrent EEG and video recording of seizures to establish the non-epileptic origin. These patients are best managed in a multi-disciplinary team with input from epileptologists, neuropsychiatrists and clinical psychologists. Cognitive-behavioural modes of treatment have met with some success.

A 68-year-old man was referred for a neurological opinion. He was complaining of slurred speech, dysphagia, limb stiffness and increasing tearfulness. A year earlier he had been referred by his GP to a local specialist with fatigue and dysarthria. On out-patient review his dysarthria had worsened and he had developed dysphagia. There was no family history of note.

On examination, he had a staring gaze, with a furrowed brow. His mental test score was normal, as were his cognitive estimates and proverbs. He was dysarthric with slow tongue movements and bilateral palmomental and snout reflexes. Cranial nerve examination was largely unremarkable apart from his eye movements. There was a decrease in voluntary up and down gaze, the latter worse than the former. Horizontal voluntary gaze was largely unimpaired. Normal eye movements were restored on eliciting oculocephalic reflexes. The patient had a festinant gait with stooped shoulders and reduced arm swing. There was impairment of postural reflexes with axial rigidity. Tone was increased in both the upper and lower limbs and there was evidence of bradykinesia. Reflexes in the upper limb were pathologically brisk with positive finger jerks. Lower limb reflexes were brisk with flexor plantar responses.

A What is the diagnosis?

B What treatment would you consider?

A Steele–Richardson–Olszewski syndrome. ✱✱✱
Cerebral Whipple's disease. ✱✱✱
Corticobasal degeneration (CBD). ✱✱

B Levodopa therapy.

Steele–Richardson–Olszewski syndrome, also known as progressive supranuclear palsy (PSP), is the combination of voluntary vertical gaze palsy (downgaze worse than upgaze) with dysarthria, axial rigidity, parkinsonism and bradyphrenia. It is a rare condition with onset between the ages of 50 and 70. It classically presents with difficulty descending stairs and reading, owing to the downgaze palsy. Dysphagia, brisk reflexes with extensor plantars and tremor may all occur. The patient becomes bedridden and anarthric after 5–7 years. Although L-dopa is used in treatment, there is little response to this therapy.

More recently, both PSP and CBD have been linked to abnormalities in tau protein. Tau, a microtubule-associated protein, is also abnormally deposited in Alzheimer's disease and other frontotemporal dementias such as Pick's disease. Originally thought to be quite separate disorders, considerable overlap in phenotype has now been identified in cases of CBD and PSP.

Cerebral Whipple's disease may also present with vertical supranucelar gaze palsy and parkinsonism. This rare disorder may occur without gastrointestinal manifestations of Whipple's disease in ~5% of cases. Co-existing dementia and psychiatric features are common. Diagnosis is possible on duodenal biopsy showing classical histology with periodic acid–Schiff (PAS)-laden macrophages in the intestinal mucosa or on a polymerase chain reaction (PCR) test on the gastric juice or CSF. Treatment is with an intravenous cephalosporin with streptomycin for 2 weeks followed by 1–2 years of oral cefixime.

A 56-year-old woman was referred with a 16-year history of watery diarrhoea, defecating 3–8 times per day. She also reported intermittent episodes of left iliac fossa pain and weight loss. Her past medical history included an appendicectomy at the age of 24 and subsequent irritable bowel syndrome. Physical examination revealed aesthenic facies with reduced skin turgor. A vesicular rash was present over the extensor surfaces of both forearms with evidence of excoriation.

The initial investigations were as follows:
Hb 10.6 g/dl, WCC 10×10^9/l, Plts 450×10^9/l, MCV 84 fl, MCH 26 pg.
Vitamin B_{12} levels 160 ng/l, serum folate 5 µg/l, red blood cell folate 112 µg/l, ferritin 4 ng/ml.

Liver function tests: bilirubin 5 µmol/l, alkaline phosphatase 180 IU/l, AST 13 IU/l, ALT 12 IU/l, total protein 55 g/l, albumin 28 g/l, globulins 27 g/l.
C-reactive protein 1 mg/l.
ESR 15 mm/h.

Urine dipstick: no protein or blood detectable.

A What is the most likely cause of the rash?

B What is the likely diagnosis?

C What further tests would you need to request to aid in diagnosis?

D What would you expect to see in the tests requested?

E How would you proceed to manage this patient?

A Dermatitis herpetiformis. ✳✳✳
   Lymphomatous skin deposits. ✳

B Coeliac disease. ✳✳✳
   Small bowel lymphoma. ✳

C Oesophagogastroduodenoscopy with duodenal biopsy. ✳✳✳
   Barium small bowel meal. ✳✳
   Anti-endomysial and reticulin antibody levels ✳✳ (anti-endomysial antibody levels of over 90% and reticulin antibody levels of over 90% in children and 60% in adults are associated with coeliac disease).
   Markers of malabsorption, e.g. iron, albumin. ✳

D Barium small bowel meal: the small bowel mucosal pattern is generally coarse and featureless, suggesting malabsorption.
   Duodenal biopsy: normal crypt architecture; chronic inflammatory infiltrate in the lamina propria consisting of lymphoid cells and plasma cells with infiltration of the enterocyte layer; total villous atrophy.

E Gluten-free diet. If the patient is unresponsive to this, she may require a lactose-free diet, steroids or investigations for possible complications such as intestinal ulceration or lymphoma.

In the absence of significant liver impairment or proteinuria, the above history of chronic diarrhoea, weight loss, decreased vitamin B_{12} and vitamin D levels (the increased alkaline phosphatase being suggestive of osteomalacia) is suggestive of a protein-losing enteropathy. Although the differential diagnosis of this is extensive, the presence of a vesicular rash over the extensor surfaces, suggestive of dermatitis herpetiformis, is indicative of coeliac disease in this age group.

   The differential diagnoses for this case include chronic small bowel infections, e.g. giardiasis, Whipple's disease, tropical sprue and blind loop syndrome; inflammatory enteropathies, e.g. Crohn's disease, eosinophilic gastroenteritis and intestinal amyloidosis; neoplasms of the small bowel, including B- and T-cell lymphomas and other gastrointestinal endocrine neoplasms, e.g. carcinoid syndrome.

A 48-year-old farmer was brought into casualty by his neighbours. He lived alone and his absence was noticed after several days. He was found unrousable in his bedroom. He was known to be a heavy drinker and several empty bottles of whisky were found in the bedroom.

On examination, he was pyrexial with a temperature of 38°C. He was jaundiced and there was a maculopapular rash present over his trunk. There was a tachycardia with a blood pressure of 90/50 mmHg. The heart sounds were normal with a loud pericardial rub audible. Chest examination revealed bibasal inspiratory crepitations. There was two-finger breadth, smooth hepatomegaly with a barely palpable spleen. Neurologically, his Glasgow coma scale (GCS) was markedly reduced; he was Kernig's negative but did have a degree of neck stiffness.

The initial investigations were as follows:
Hb 14.5 g/dl, WCC 13.6 × 10^9/l (90% neutrophils), Plts 120 × 10^9/l.
Sodium 130 mmol/l, potassium 5.0 mmol/l, urea 26 mmol/l, creatinine 340 µmol/l
Bicarbonate 16 mmol/l, bilirubin 80 µmol/l, albumin 30 g/l, ALT 78 IU/l
Alkaline phosphatase 740 IU/l.

Urine dipstick: protein + +, blood + +.
Four hours after starting treatment, his temperature rose and he became flushed and tachycardic.

A What is the likely diagnosis?

B What further tests would you carry out to confirm your diagnosis?

C How would you treat this patient?

D What is the cause of his deterioration on treatment?

A Weil's disease. ✱✱✱
Fulminant viral hepatitis with hepatic encephalopathy and functional renal failure. ✱✱
Alcohol-induced hepatic encephalopathy with infection. ✱
Other infections: Epstein–Barr virus (EBV)/cytomegalovirus (CMV)/Legionnaire's/Brucellosis. ✱

B Blood culture. ✱✱✱
Urine culture and microscopy for leptospires. ✱✱
Lumbar puncture with microscopy and culture. ✱✱
Serology for leptospirosis. ✱✱
Hepatitis A/B/C serology. ✱
Serology for EBV/CMV/*Legionnella*/*Brucella*. ✱
Electroencephalogram (EEG). ✱

C High-dose intravenous benzylpenicillin within the first 4–7 days
Supportive treatment for renal and liver failure; may require dialysis

D Jarisch–Herxheimer reaction.

This is a typical picture for Weil's disease. The illness is caused by a spirochaete, the main reservoir being thought to be rodents. People who work in close vicinity to rodents or other small mammals are at increased risk, e.g. there is a high rate of seropositivity for previous leptospirosis infections among British dairy farmers.

The incubation period of infection is 7–12 days and the disease may present as Weil's disease with jaundice and multi-organ failure or may present with a milder anicteric form. Both have a biphasic course, with an initial septic phase (involving rigors, abdominal pain, a typical rash, acute hepatorenal failure and arthritis) followed by an immune phase (incorporating meningitis, uveitis, fever and various neurological sequelae, including paralysis and cranial nerve palsies).

In the first 10 days of illness, blood and CSF may yield leptospires. After this period, urine and serology for leptospires become positive. CSF usually shows normal glucose, with elevated protein and a lymphocytic or neutrophilic pleiocytosis. The Jarisch–Herxheimer reaction is due to the massive release of endotoxin when a large number of organisms are killed. It was most often described in the treatment of syphilis, and can be fatal.

A 23-year-old woman, in her first pregnancy, presented at 21 weeks' gestation. Her pregnancy had been complicated by mild systolic hypertension. She was referred to the medical team on call with a gradual onset of a fronto-occipital headache, which had persisted for 4 hours in association with vomiting, unsteadiness and inability to stand. On examination, she was restless and manifestly photophobic. There was no rash. She was afebrile, had a left homonymous hemianopia, increased cervical tone and was Kernig's sign positive. There was full power in the limbs, in association with normal reflexes and flexor plantar responses.

Her ESR was 10 mm/h and full blood count showed Hb 12.2 g/dl, WCC 3.7×10^9/l and platelets 370×10^9/l. Her family gave a history of a similar episode 8 months earlier which presented with sudden headache and transitory left-sided weakness resolving over 3 months. She was a known migraineur.

A What is the diagnosis?

B Where is the probable site of the lesion?

C What investigations are necessary?

A Intracerebral bleed from right hemisphere arteriovenous malformation. *******
Bleed into right hemispheric tumour. ******
Spontaneous intracerebral haemorrhage. ******
Migraine. *****

B Right occipito-parietal area, involving the right optic tract.

C CT brain. *******
Four-vessel cerebral angiogram via femoral catheterization. *******
Lumbar puncture if scan shows no evidence of intracerebral bleed. ******
Magnetic resonance angiography (MRA). ******
Angiography. *****

Most arteriovenous malformations have become symptomatic before the age of 40 years. The commonest presentation is as a spontaneous intracranial haemorrhage, mostly intracerebral, although intraventricular, subdural or subarachnoid haemorrhage may also occur. There may be an association with hypertension and pregnancy. Arteriovenous malformations may also present as epilepsy, a focal mass lesion or cerebral ischaemia. The degree of neck stiffness in this case implies the presence of blood in the CSF, making a bleed into a tumour less likely. The past medical history of a similar headache with left-sided weakness is more suggestive of a previous bleed from this lesion.

The presentation is not entirely incompatible with migraine, although the amaurosis that can result tends to be part of the visual aura and does not produce a homonymous hemianopic defect.

The choice of formal angiography vs. MRA is debatable. Angiography carries a 1–2% risk of stroke or other serious morbidity in those who are over 60; the amount of blood present after an intracerebral bleed may prevent accurate identification of the lesion and may defer angiography to an elective examination up to 6 weeks later. However, angiography remains the examination of choice given the above history as a neurosurgeon would be unlikely to operate on the basis of MRA alone.

A 50-year-old man presented with a 6-month history of fatigue, weight loss and increased swelling of his legs below the knees. He had noticed increased difficulty in masticating and swallowing his food recently. He had no previous hospital admissions and was taking no regular medications. There was no relevant family history. On examination, his pulse was 80/min, regular, blood pressure 120/90 mmHg (lying flat), 90/70 mmHg (standing). Cardiac auscultation was unremarkable. Chest examination revealed bilateral pleural effusions. Abdominal examination was normal. There was bilateral wasting of the thenar eminence with some weakness of abductor pollicis brevis. In addition, there was associated sensory loss over the thenar eminence and the palmar surfaces of the index and middle fingers. A purpuric rash was present on his forehead with prominent ecchymoses around his eyes.

The initial investigations were as follows:
Hb 12.2 g/dl, WCC 10×10^9/l, Plts 200×10^9/l.
Chest radiograph: cardiac enlargement, pulmonary venous congestion.
ECG: sinus rhythm, low voltage complexes, QS pattern in leads V1–3.

A What is the diagnosis?

B What further investigations would you request?

A Primary amyloidosis with cardiac involvement. ✱✱✱
Vasculitis with right heart failure. ✱

B Rectal biopsy. ✱✱✱
Endomyocardial biopsy. ✱✱
Transthoracic echocardiogram. ✱✱
Serum protein electrophoresis and early morning urine for Bence-Jones proteins. ✱✱
Urea and electrolytes. ✱
ESR, CRP and vasculitic serology. ✱

Amyloidosis may be primary, secondary, familial or senile. Cardiac involvement is commonest in the primary form, which is characterized by the deposition of an excess of a monoclonal immunoglobulin light chain protein. The clinical presentation may be typically as described above, with predominant right heart failure due to diastolic dysfunction, autonomic neuropathy (producing postural hypotension), carpal tunnel syndrome, pleural effusions, a purpuric facial rash accompanied by periorbital ecchymoses and macroglossia.

Familial amyloidosis may be subdivided into four types on the basis of the protein product deposited. Types I and II have mutations of plasma transthyretin. Type I involves the heart and kidney with an autonomic and sensorimotor neuropathy. Type II involves the heart with additional carpal tunnel syndrome. Type III involves deposition of an abnormal fragment of apolipoprotein A1 and involves the kidney with additional peptic ulceration and a sensorimotor neuropathy. Type IV involves deposition of gelsolin, an actin-binding protein found in plasma and leucocytes. Presentation is with corneal clouding due to a fine network of amyloid filaments, referred to as lattice corneal dystrophy. In addition, progressive cranial neuropathies can develop, leading to a bulbar presentation with baggy skin over an atrophic facies. A mild peripheral neuropathy may be present.

A 30-year-old man was admitted with a history of malaise, anorexia and fatigue. His previous history was unremarkable apart from trauma sustained during the course of a road traffic accident 10 years previously whilst working abroad. He underwent surgery, and blood transfusion was necessary.

His GP had organized some blood tests and the results of these precipitated his referral to the out-patients' clinic:
Hb 12.5 g/dl, WCC 6×10^9/l, Plts 170×10^9/l.
Blood film: reactive lymphocytes.
Bilirubin 18 µmol/l, alkaline phosphatase 71 IU/l, AST 239 IU/l, ALT 368 IU/l, total protein, albumin and globulin levels normal.
Hepatitis B serology: anti-hepatitis B surface, core and 'e' antigen antibodies positive; hepatitis B surface antigen and 'e' antigen negative.
Hepatitis A antibody negative.

A What additional tests are necessary?

B What is the likely diagnosis?

A Hepatitis C RNA polymerase chain reaction test. ✱✱✱
Liver biopsy. ✱✱
HIV test. ✱

B Hepatitis C consequent to the transfusion of infected blood. ✱✱✱
HIV infection secondary to blood transfusion. ✱

The blood film suggests a reactive lymphocytic response, possibly to a viral infection. The patient already reveals prior exposure to hepatitis B (although he is not a carrier). His liver function tests suggest hepatocellular damage. Hepatitis C has therefore to be excluded, particularly in view of his previous blood transfusion. Interferon α produces cure in a number of cases.

A 49-year-old man presented with a 6-month history of episodes of shaking of his arms and legs, weakness and syncope. He was usually drowsy in the mornings until he had breakfast and then would usually function well until before lunchtime, when he would invariably have one of his attacks, particularly if lunch was delayed. There was no incontinence or tongue biting during these attacks. He was not taking any medications and alcohol consumption was negligible. Physical examination was unremarkable, except for the presence of obesity.

The results of his initial investigations were as follows:
Urea and electrolytes normal.
Random glucose normal.
Full blood count and liver function normal.

A What further investigations would you request in order to aid diagnosis?

B What is the likely diagnosis?

C What treatment is necessary?

A 48–72 h fasting glucose assessments correlated with a symptom diary. ✻✻✻
Concomitant insulin, C-peptide and glucose levels. ✻✻✻
CT scan of the abdomen. ✻✻
Urinary screen for sulphonylurea abuse. ✻✻
EEG. ✻
24-hour cardiac tape. ✻

B Insulinoma. ✻✻✻
Therapeutic or factitious use of insulin or oral hypoglycaemic. ✻✻
Rare extra-pancreatic tumours. ✻
Epilepsy. ✻
Non-epileptic attacks. ✻
Cardiac arrhythmia. ✻

C The initial management of insulinoma includes taking regular meals with a high carbohydrate content. Surgical removal of the tumour may be feasible in some patients. The medical treatment includes diazoxide, a thiazide diuretic with potent diabetogenic potential (available on a named patient basis). Subcutaneous injections of octreotide may be used to suppress insulin production. Streptozotocin, an intravenously administered chemotherapeutic agent that is toxic to the pancreatic β-cells, is also available (but the patient is liable to be rendered permanently diabetic with this). Refractory cases of hypoglycaemia may require treatment with steroids and growth hormone to elevate the blood sugar levels. In patients with hepatic metastases, hepatic embolization may be very effective.

The history presented is typical of that of a patient with insulinoma, with presentation in late middle age and symptoms that are relieved by eating. A variety of neurological manifestations may occur, including fits and diplopia. The presence of hyperinsulinaemia in the presence of fasting and hypoglycaemia suggests this diagnosis, although retroperitoneal fibrosarcoma and mesothelioma may also secrete insulin-like growth factors under these conditions. Exogenous insulin administration is excluded by a low C-peptide level. Patients taking sulphonylureas will have raised insulin and C-peptide levels. Abuse of these agents may only be excluded by performing a urinary sulphonylurea screen. Malignant insulinomas (10% of the total) have usually metastasized to the liver at the time of diagnosis. Streptozotocin may be used here. Somatostatin infusion or subcutaneous injections may be helpful in some patients.

A 60-year-old woman presented with a 2-month history of swollen eyes and weakness. She had been prescribed steroids for an exacerbation of her pre-existing asthma. This had also decreased the swelling surrounding her eyes. On examination, she had periorbital swelling and was weak, especially in the proximal musculature of the upper and lower limb. A lump was palpable in her left breast.

Her investigations were as follows:
Creatinine kinase 20 IU/l.
Skin biopsy: epidermal atrophy.
Muscle biopsy: dense mononuclear infiltrate with some fibres exhibiting degenerative changes.

A What is the diagnosis?

B What further tests are necessary to confirm the diagnosis?

A Dermatomyositis with probable underlying breast carcinoma. ✱✱✱
Dermatomyositis. ✱✱
Polymyositis. ✱
Paraneoplastic myopathy. ✱

B EMG. ✱✱✱
Mammography. ✱✱
Biopsy of breast lump. ✱✱
ESR. ✱

Muscle pain, tenderness and weakness accompanied by the characteristic facial discoloration, periorbital swelling and Gottron's papules would suggest a diagnosis of dermatomyositis. The creatinine kinase, serum glutamate oxaloacetate transaminase (SGOT) and aldolase may not necessarily be elevated, although they are often found to be so. Skin biopsy in this condition is non-specific, although skin changes can be more disabling than the muscle weakness in longstanding dermatomyositis. Muscle biopsy is more useful, showing muscle fibre degeneration, necrosis and a perivascular cellular infiltrate consisting mainly of lymphocytes and macrophages. The cellular infiltrate is of B-cell lineage in dermatomyositis and of T-cell lineage in polymyositis. There is said to be an association between dermatomyositis and malignancy, probably in the region of 10–20%. The types of neoplasia most often seen include breast, lung, ovary and stomach. A normal ESR should exclude polymyalgia rheumatica: the CK in this condition is usually normal and muscle biopsy may show non-specific type 2 fibre atrophy. EMG in dermatomyositis shows myopathic features together with signs of muscle hyperirritability: small, polyphasic muscle action potentials are seen with increased insertional activity, fibrillations and on occasion, positive sharp waves.

A 70-year-old woman presented with a 3-week history of increasing weakness of her right leg. She had tried a variety of herbal remedies without improvement. Her right leg had been weaker than the left for many years due to a slipped disc 10 years earlier. She was an ex-smoker and an occasional drinker.

On examination she had a left homonymous upper quadrantinopia. The fundi were not well visualized due to bilateral cataracts. In the upper limb there were signs of a right-sided hemiparesis with increased tone, brisk reflexes with finger jerks and mild pyramidal weakness. In the lower limb, the tone was increased in the right leg with decreased strength in hip and knee flexion, and more marked decrease in plantar flexion and dorsiflexion of the ankle, flexion of the big toe and eversion of the ankle. The knee jerk was brisk on the right with an absent ankle jerk. The left plantar was flexor and the right plantar was absent.

Her investigations were as follows:
Hb 12.3 g/dl, total WCC 10.0×10^9/l, Plts 505×10^9/l.
Sodium 138 mmol/l, potassium 4.4 mmol/l, urea 4.3 mmol/l, creatinine 67 µmol/l.
LFTs normal.
CRP 10 mg/l.
Chest radiograph showed a mass at the right hilum.

A Explain this patient's neurological signs.

B What further test would you carry out to achieve a diagnosis?

A Kernohan's notch phenomenon due to a metastasis from the bronchus to the right temporal lobe. *******
Right temporal lobe and left parietal lobe multiple metastases. ******
Right-sided L5/S1 disc protrusion. *****

B MRI brain. *******
CT brain. ******
CT chest with fine needle aspiration biopsy. ******

The left upper homonymous quadrantinopia is suggestive of a right temporal lesion impinging on the inferior fibres of the right optic radiation. Tumours in this area can cause compression of the contralateral cerebral peduncle, and hence corticospinal fibres, against the tentorium. This leads to hemiparesis on the same side as the temporal lesion: a phenomenon known as Kernohan's notch sign; compression of the III cranial nerve can also occur at this level. The additional signs in the right leg, with the absent plantar reflex, the absent ankle jerk and the weakness in plantar flexion, can all be explained by the past history of an L5/S1 disc lesion causing additional lower motor neurone signs. This patient may also have multiple metastases causing bilateral neurological signs.

A middle-aged man was referred with a history of diarrhoea. He had noted loose motions for the preceding 3 months at a frequency of five times per day. The motions contained both blood and mucus. He had lost weight and his appetite was poor. There was no relevant past medical history. On examination, there were no specific findings.

Investigation yielded the following information:
Hb 10.1 g/dl, Plts 1000×10^9/l, WCC 18×10^9/l: neutrophils 70%, lymphocytes 18%, monocytes 11%, eosinophils 1%.
Stool microscopy and culture: no organisms visualized or grown.
Barium meal and follow-through: normal.
Colonoscopy: perianal fissure; distorted ulcerated rectum.
Histology: chronic inflammation of the lamina propria in the ascending, transverse and descending colon. Florid chronic active procto-colitis.

A What is the diagnosis?

B What are the possible treatment options?

A Crohn's colitis. ★★★

B Medical: steroids, antibiotics, 5-aminosalicylic acid drugs, azathioprine (see below).
Surgical: strictureplasty or bowel resection.

Crohn's disease is an inflammation of the bowel which may occur at any site between the mouth and the anus. Although it is characterized by a granulomatous inflammation, granulomata are in fact only present at biopsy in two-thirds of cases. The principal presenting feature is diarrhoea, which may contain blood (particularly in more distal disease). Weight loss and abdominal pain may also be evident. Distal disease is also associated with perianal disease (fistulae, fissures and abscesses), as in this case.

The principal mode of treatment for active Crohn's disease is the use of steroids. Antibiotics, e.g. metronidazole may also be useful, particularly when secondary infection is believed to exist. Sulphasalazine may be limited in its usefulness, since it may release the active drug, 5-aminosalicylic acid, into the large bowel, thereby missing small bowel disease. Slow-release mesalazine and olsalazine, however, also act in the small bowel. Unlike ulcerative colitis, maintaining remission for Crohn's colitis is comparatively difficult. Azathioprine is effective in selected patient groups. Ineffectiveness of medical therapy alone may require the use of surgery, e.g. surgical resection of the terminal ileum with an ileo-colic anastomosis or strictureplasty.

A 23-year-old woman was referred to the medical registrar on call from the psychiatric department. She had been admitted that day for assessment of her depressive illness and had been noted to be hypertensive. Her past medical history was unremarkable, although she had recently consulted her GP concerning her dysmenorrhoea. On examination, she was noted to be obese and had facial hair and acne. She had bruising on her shins and a cut on her hand, which had been slow to heal. Her blood pressure was 170/120 mmHg and although no retinal abnormalities were noted she had proteinuria and glycosuria.

The results of initial investigations are shown:
Hb 14 g/dl.
ESR 5 mm/h.
Sodium 135 mmol/l, potassium 2.9 mmol/l, urea 7 mmol/l.

Plasma steroid and adrenocorticotrophic hormone (ACTH)

Day	Time	Cortisol (nmol/l)	ACTH (pg/ml)
1	0100	500	180
2	Midnight	470	175
2	0900	370	175
3 Dexamethasone, 0.5 mg, qds for 48 h			
5	0800	400	

Insulin-induced hypoglycaemia test

Time (min)	Glucose (mmol/l)	Growth hormone (ng/ml)	Cortisol (nmol/l)	ACTH (pg/ml)
1	3.6	3.9	1225	130
2	3.6	2.4	1200	
15	2.8			
30	1.6	6.3	1150	
45	2.4			145
60	3.1	2.1	1200	
90	3.5	1.3	1225	
120	3.7	0.8	1150	

A What information is obtained from the plasma cortisol and ACTH data?

B What is the likely diagnosis?

C What is the differential diagnosis based on the results of the low-dose dexamethasone suppression test?

D What further test is needed?

A There are elevated levels of plasma cortisol and ACTH. The expected diurnal variation in the plasma cortisol is absent. In normal individuals cortisol is undetectable at midnight, provided the patient is asleep.

B Cushing's syndrome. ✻✻✻
Cushing's disease. ✻✻
Alcohol abuse. ✻
Depression. ✻

Cushing's disease implies a pituitary cause which is unlikely given the hypokalaemia (which is worst with ectopic ACTH) and the very high ACTH. ACTH levels are usually marginally raised with pituitary-dependent Cushing's disease.

An ACTH-dependent hypersecretion of cortisol may occur in cases of alcohol abuse (pseudo-Cushing's syndrome) and depressive psychosis. The insulin sensitivity test can help to distinguish between these patients and those with Cushing's disease. The normal response to hypoglycaemia is a rise in the growth hormone and cortisol levels. This response is preserved in alcohol abuse and depression. In Cushing's disease, there is no concomitant rise in the plasma cortisol.

C Cushing's syndrome which may be due to pituitary-dependant Cushing's disease or ectopic ACTH release. An adrenal adenoma is excluded by the high ACTH levels.

D High-dose dexamethasone suppression test: 2 mg dexamethasone is administered 6-hourly for 48 hours. A fall in the plasma cortisol concentration of 50% would suggest pituitary-dependant Cushing's disease. No such change will occur in ectopic ACTH release.

A 16-year-old girl was referred to psychiatric out-patients, with a change in her personality. She had been born in India and had been well until the age of 10, when she began to suffer from recurrent vomiting and weight loss. Her problems continued over the years, and at the age of 12 she was admitted to hospital for treatment of suspected anorexia nervosa.

When she was 15, her family moved to England. Over the course of the subsequent year her family noted a change in her temperament; she became irritable and prone to temper tantrums. Her school work deteriorated markedly, and she achieved poorer GCSE grades than predicted. Her school teachers found her a difficult pupil and suggested psychiatric evaluation.

On examination, she was prone to drooling and had slurred speech. Cardiac and respiratory examinations were unremarkable. On abdominal examination, she had a three-finger breadth liver and a palpable spleen. Neurologically, there was dystonic posturing of her right hand, and there was lead-pipe rigidity in all limbs. She had bilateral reduced arm swing and bradykinesia. The reflexes and plantar responses were normal. There were no gross cerebellar features.

She was referred for a medical opinion, with the following investigations:
Sodium 130 mmol/l, potassium 4.2 mmol/l, urea 1.2 mmol/l, creatinine 90 μmol/l.
Bilirubin 30 μmol/l, albumin 32 g/l, GGT 85 IU/l, AST 62 IU/l, alkaline phosphatase 220 IU/l.
Hb 9.8 g/dl, WCC 9×10⁹/l, Plts 320×10⁹/l, MCV 102 fl.
PT 16 s.
Coombs' test negative.

A What is the likely underlying diagnosis?

B Suggest a cause of her anaemia.

C What further tests would you carry out to confirm your diagnosis?

D How would you manage this patient?

After 3 months of treatment, the patient was reviewed in out-patients. A repeat full blood count showed the following result:
Hb 9.2 g/dl, WCC 2.2×10⁹/l, Plts 80×10⁹/l, MCV 95 fl.

E How would you explain the above result?

A Wilson's disease. ✳✳✳
Acaeruloplasminaemia. ✳✳
Hallervorden–Spatz disease. ✳
Hypoprebetalipoproteinaemia, acanthocytosis and retinitis pigmentosa (HARP) syndrome. ✳
Neuroacanthocytosis. ✳
Dentatorubropallidoluysian atrophy (DRPLA). ✳

B Hypersplenism leading to extravascular haemolysis.

C Slit-lamp examination for Kayser–Fleischer (KF) rings. ✳✳✳
Measurement of free serum copper, total serum copper, serum caeruloplasmin. ✳✳✳
24-hour urinary copper. ✳
MRI brain. ✳✳

D D-penicillamine.
Trientine.

E This is a likely side-effect of penicillamine treatment leading to leucopenia and thrombocytopenia. This drug may also cause aplastic anaemia, SLE and immune complex nephritis.

The association of hepatic dysfunction with neurological signs, sparing the sensory system, should always make one consider the diagnosis of Wilson's disease. The detection of KF rings may require slit-lamp examination in patients with pigmented irises; their presence is not pathognomonic of Wilson's disease, but their absence makes the diagnosis very unlikely. The rings are due to the deposition of copper deep in Descemet's membrane, and start at the upper limbus of the cornea, eventually joining up with deposition around the lower limbus to complete the ring. They tend to disappear with effective therapy and may reappear with a relapse of disease.

Wilson's has a wide age presentation, and can often present to psychiatrists with change in personality. Presentation may also be with haemolytic crises due to the hypersplenism. Neurological features are widespread and include drooling, slurred speech, bats-wing tremor, akinetic rigidity, dystonia and chorea. Copper deposition in the abdominal viscera gives rise to hepatosplenomegaly, and renal deposition may result in renal tubular acidosis, mild proteinuria and glycosuria. A liver biopsy may show hepatitis and cirrhosis, with increased dry weight of copper/wet weight liver. CT scan of the brain may show hypodensity of the basal ganglia with cortical atrophy.

The remaining diagnoses outlined above may produce a similar neurological picture with dystonia and bulbar extra-pyramidal features. None of them produce liver abnormalities and in this particular case are much less likely.

Treatment of Wilson's disease involves reducing copper intake through dietary means (difficult to achieve in practice) or reducing gastrointestinal absorption with zinc sulphate. D-penicillamine and trientine both act as copper-chelating agents. The former agent should be given after checking the electrolytes and full blood count, in view of its possible side-effects.

A 28-year-old woman presented with a 3-day history of an itchy rash. She had endured a sore throat for 2 weeks for which her GP prescribed a course of antibiotics. In addition, she gave a 1-week history of a dry cough with shortness of breath on exertion. On examination, she had cold sores on her upper lip. There were target lesions present on her forearms, legs and feet. The throat was inflamed with enlarged tonsils. Her chest was clinically clear.

A What condition does she have?

B Give the likely cause in this particular case.

A Erythema multiforme.

B Herpes simplex virus. ✱✱✱
Mycoplasma pneumoniae pneumonia. ✱✱✱
Streptococcal sore throat. ✱✱

Erythema multiforme is a rash consisting of symmetrically distributed erythematous papules in concentric ring patterns. It can occur 1–2 weeks after *Herpes simplex* virus infections (as suggested by this patient's cold sore). Her dry cough and shortness of breath may also have suggested underlying *Mycoplasma pneumoniae* pneumonia, which is another cause of this skin eruption.

A 69-year-old woman was referred to the out-patients' clinic with a 10-year history of postprandial diarrhoea, occurring up to four times per day. The stools were described as pale and difficult to flush away from the toilet basin. There was no blood loss per rectum and no history of weight loss or abdominal pain. In addition, there was no history of foreign travel. The clinical examination was unremarkable.

Her initial investigations were as follows:
Hb 11 g/dl, WCC 5.4×10^9/l, Plts 150×10^9/l, MCV 110 fl.

Bilirubin 6 μmol/l, alkaline phosphatase 70 IU/l, AST 20 IU/l, ALT 25 IU/l, total protein 50 g/l, albumin 28 g/l, globulins 22 g/l, calcium 1.98 mmol/l.

Schilling test
Part one: ^{57}Co-B$_{12}$ excretion 0.3% (urine volume 1300 ml)
Part two (with addition of intrinsic factor). ^{57}Co-B$_{12}$ excretion 1.5% (urine volume 1300 ml)

Hydrogen breath test

	H_2 (p.p.m.)
Fasting	5
Postprandial	
1 hour	20
2 hours	54
3 hours	74
4 hours	50
5 hours	22

A What is the cause of the macrocytosis?

B What conclusions may be obtained from the hydrogen breath test?

C What further tests are required?

A Vitamin B_{12} deficiency secondary to malabsorption. ✳✳✳
Vitamin B_{12} deficiency secondary to pernicious anaemia. ✳✳

The Schilling test confirms that this is due to malabsorption, since the initial excretion of radio-labelled vitamin B_{12} is subnormal (less than 10%) and this is not correctable in part two of the test by the administration of intrinsic factor. In addition, there is a subnormal level of plasma albumin.

B There is an excess of hydrogen exhaled, confirming the presence of bacterial overgrowth.
The hydrogen breath test is a useful device by which the presence of bacterial over-growth may be investigated. It consists of the administration of glucose with the detection of exhaled hydrogen. In the presence of bacterial over-growth, excess hydrogen is exhaled (>20 p.p.m.). The timing of the peak may correlate with the site of bacterial colonization, i.e. the small bowel peak occurs prior to the large bowel one. In practice, the extrapolation of such information from this feature is unreliable.

C Part three of the Schilling test ✳✳✳: urinary ^{57}Co-B_{12} excretion following a course of antibiotics. If this remains low, even after antibiotic treatment, disease of the terminal ileum should be suspected, e.g. Crohn's disease.
Small bowel follow-through. ✳
Aspiration of secretions from the small bowel for culture. ✳

Stagnation of intestinal contents is the substrate for bacterial over-growth:
- small bowel diverticulae
- the presence of bowel fistulae (due to Crohn's disease or malignancy)
- stagnant loops following surgery
- abnormal bowel motility
   Treatment consists of correction of the specific nutritional deficiency, e.g. vitamin B_{12} replacement and antibiotic therapy.

A 52-year-old solicitor was admitted through casualty with a 1-month history of increasing shortness of breath. He had been intermittently pyrexial during this time but had a non-productive cough. He had lost his appetite and half a stone in weight. He had had two courses of antibiotics from his GP without effect. In the past he had had a bout of pneumococcal pneumonia confirmed on blood cultures; he had otherwise been a fit individual. He was a lifelong non-smoker who had always been single. He was not taking any medication and was allergic to penicillin and cotrimoxazole.

On examination he was pyrexial and emaciated. There were umbilicated lesions present on his face and hands. Cardiovascular, abdominal and neurological examinations, including fundoscopy, were entirely normal. Respiratory examination revealed vesicular breath sounds with fine bibasal inspiratory crepitations.

Investigations on admission are shown:
Hb 10.9 g/dl, total WCC 3.9 × 10^9/l, Plts 254 × 10^9/l.
Sodium 127 mmol/l, potassium 4.3 mmol/l, bicarbonate 26 mmol/l, urea 3.5 mmol/l, creatinine 62 µmol/l, glucose 5.7 mmol/l, albumin 22 g/l, alkaline phosphatase 50 IU/l, ALT 17 IU/l, bilirubin 11 µmol/l.
Blood gases on air: pH 7.5, P_{CO_2} 3 kPa, P_{O_2} 10.2 kPa, standard HCO_3^- 22 mmol/l.
Base excess + 0.2, saturation 96%.

Chest radiograph: interstitial shadowing across both mid-zones with basal and apical sparing, and bilateral cyst formation.

A What is the most likely cause of this man's breathing problems?

B What is the likely underlying diagnosis?

C What further tests would you perform?

D How would you treat this man and what are the hazards of treatment?

A *Pneumocystis carinii* pneumonia (PCP). ✱✱✱
Atypical pneumonia. ✱

B Acute presentation of AIDS.

PCP often has a very characteristic chest radiograph appearance, with mid-zone, interstitial shadowing sparing the apices and bases. Cyst formation is said to occur in up to 10%. The illness often has an insidious onset, with a chronic cough and mucoid sputum. Fever occurs in the majority but shortness of breath is a relatively late sign. Rhales are audible on auscultation in severe cases. Blood gases typically show hypoxia with hypocarbia, and lung function shows a drop in carbon monoxide transfer factor (TLCO) to less than 70% predicted. Serum LDH is elevated in up to 90%. The disease typically occurs in the setting of HIV disease at a CD4 count of 50–75 cells/mm^3.

Florid facial molluscum contagiosum is closely correlated with HIV disease. This man actually presented with PCP as his first presentation of underlying HIV — this is an AIDS-defining illness.

C Bronchoalveolar lavage with direct/indirect immunofluorescent or methenamine silver staining for cysts. ✱✱✱
HIV test after counselling. ✱✱
Blood cultures. ✱
Antibody titres for atypical pneumonia. ✱

D Intravenous pentamidine as allergic to cotrimoxazole.
High-dose oxygen.

When using pentamidine one must monitor renal function, blood pressure and blood glucose (side-effects include hypotension and hypoglycaemia).

A 36-year-old woman was referred for an out-patients' appointment. Her GP wrote that this usually punctual woman had turned up for her surgery appointment 2 hours late. Her sense of dress was unusually eccentric. She seemed vague and easily distractible, but answered all the GP's questions accurately.

A few days later the GP had been called to the woman's house by a concerned friend. The friend had called to visit but had initially been denied access by the woman who shouted obscenities through the letter-box at him.

Examination in the out-patients' clinic was grossly unremarkable apart from lack of pulsation of the retinal veins bilaterally on fundoscopy. Mental state test revealed a poor short-term memory and difficulty with serial sevens. Cognitive estimates were poor and proverb translation was literal. Visuospatial functioning was well preserved with no evidence of apraxia.

A What is the likely diagnosis?

B List the tests and the order in which you would carry them out.

C What drugs would you consider starting the patient on?

A Frontal lobe syndrome (FLS) secondary to a space-occupying lesion. ✱✱✱
Cerebral venous sinus thrombosis. ✱✱✱
Fronto-temporal dementia secondary to disorder of tau protein, e.g. Alzheimer's disease (AD) or Pick's disease. ✱✱
Parenchymal brain disorder due to infection or inflammation. ✱

B MRI brain with gadolinium enhancement. ✱✱✱
MRI brain. ✱✱
Magnetic resonance venography. ✱✱
If no evidence of space-occupying lesion and if there is adequate space around the quadrigeminal cisterns then consider lumbar puncture. ✱✱
Bloods including ESR, CRP, serum angiotensin converting enzyme (ACE), autoantibodies, vasculitic serology, anticardiolipin antibody, syphilis serology, lupus anticoagulant, clotting. ✱

C Dexamethasone to reduce intracranial pressure.
Phenytoin as antiepileptic prophylaxis in the presence of a space-occupying lesion.
If cerebral venous sinus thrombosis then for intravenous heparin and warfarinization.
If thought to be dementia of Alzheimer type, then consider aricept (donepezil).

This 36-year-old patient has presented with a coarsening of her personality with forgetfulness. Examination reveals her to perform poorly in tests sensitive to frontal lobe function, e.g. cognitive estimates and translation of proverbs. She has no other focal neurology but had early changes of papilloedema with lack of pulsation of retinal veins.

Raised intracranial pressure and a frontal lobe syndrome in this age group is most suggestive of a frontal lobe tumour, either a meningioma or a glioma. Alternatively, cerebral venous sinus can present with a variety of neurological symptoms and signs, including a dementing process, and should be excluded. Underlying causes include pro-thrombotic conditions, e.g. anti-phospholipid syndrome. An infective or inflammatory CSF process may also produce raised intracerebral pressure from high CSF protein levels causing a block to CSF flow from the foramina of Luschka and Magendie or blockage of the arachnoid granulations.

Obviously, if a lesion is seen on the CT scan not all the possible blood tests suggested above would need to be carried out. The lumbar puncture has to be carried out after the scan to avoid coning of the cerebellar tonsils in the presence of raised intracranial pressure. The lumbar puncture may give further useful information if an infectious/inflammatory aetiology is under consideration. Note that oligoclonal bands are not pathognomonic for multiple sclerosis and are found in, for example, neurosarcoidosis and cerebral Lyme disease.

The classification of fronto-temporal dementia has been updated in recent years due to the discovery of mutations and phosphorylation abnormalities in tau protein. Tau is one of the microtubule-associated proteins.

A 70-year-old man was admitted to casualty having been found unconscious. His GP's letter detailed a history of gradual deterioration over the course of the previous 6 months, accelerating over the winter months, until he was almost house-bound. On examination, his temperature was 35°C, his pulse was 48/min, blood pressure 120/90 mmHg and he was breathing spontaneously. He was unconscious, had coarse features, and was pale and balding with dry skin. Neurological assessment revealed generalized hypotonia, the reflexes being difficult to elicit. The remainder of the examination was unremarkable.

The results of initial investigations were as follows:
ECG: sinus bradycardia, low voltage complexes in the limb leads with prominent 'u' waves.
Hb 11 g/dl, WCC 11 × 10⁹/l, Plts 150 × 10⁹/l, MCV 100 fl.
Sodium 129 mmol/l, potassium 4.8 mmol/l, bicarbonate 27 mmol/l, urea 7 mmol/l, creatinine 130 µmol/l, random blood glucose 6 mmol/l.

A What is the most likely diagnosis?

B How would you manage this patient?

A Myxoedema coma. ✳✳
Schmidt's syndrome. ✳

B This is a medical emergency with quoted mortality rates as high as 50% in established coma. The management consists of taking baseline blood tests such as full blood count, urea, electrolytes, glucose, arterial blood gases, cortisol, thyroid function tests and serum amylase.

The current practice centres on giving intravenous ʟ-triiodothyronine sodium (liothyronine sodium) at doses of 5–20 μg b.d. initially, although it can be given up to 4-hourly, until a sustained clinical response has been obtained. The intravenous T3 may be administered orally once the patient is conscious and later changed to T4 100–200 μg/day. As hypothyroidism with coexistent Addison's disease **(Schmidt's syndrome)** is a possibility, it has also been practice to give intravenous hydrocortisone and fluids. The hydrocortisone can then be stopped once the admission cortisol level has been shown to be normal. Administration of thyroxine to a patient with Addison's disease may result in an Addisonian crisis. Hypoxia or hypercapnoea must be treated aggressively, with ventilation if necessary.

This diagnosis should always be considered in an elderly unconscious patient, particularly during the winter months. An insidious onset is frequently the case. This patient also has many of the clinical features of hypothyroidism, including hypothermia, hair/skin changes and bradycardia. A prolonged relaxation phase to the reflexes is often, but not invariably present. The presence of hyponatraemia, a macrocytosis and the low-voltage ECG would tend to corroborate the clinical diagnosis.

A 50-year-old merchant seaman was referred to the medical out-patients' clinic with a history of effort dyspnoea over the preceding 6 months in association with exertional retrosternal chest pain. He also described orthopnoea and paroxysmal nocturnal dyspnoea. He had suffered from rheumatic fever as a child. Whilst sailing in the Far East 15 years previously he had been treated for gonorrhoea with antibiotics. There was a history of arthritis of the back and hips. He was a smoker of 20 cigarettes per day. On examination, he was 5 feet tall with a stooping posture. He had a pulse rate of 96/min, BP 170/60 with a collapsing carotid pulse and an audible early diastolic murmur along the right sternal edge. There were no skin, skeletal or neurological findings of note.

The results of his initial investigations are shown below:
Chest radiograph: cardiomegaly, calcification of the ascending aorta and aortic arch, both of which appeared aneurysmal.
ECG: atrial flutter with variable AV block, left bundle branch block.
ESR 23 mm/h.
Hb 14 g/dl.

A What further tests are necessary in the further assessment of this patient?

B What is the most likely diagnosis?

A Transthoracic echocardiogram. ✱✱✱
Cardiac catheterization. ✱✱
Syphilis serology: treponemal haemagglutination test, VDRL and FTA-ABS test. ✱✱
X-rays back/hips. ✱
Rheumatoid factor (may be falsely positive in syphilis). ✱

B Luetic aortitis and aortic regurgitation. ✱✱✱
Angina pectoris possibly due to ischaemic heart disease or luetic coronary osteal stenosis. ✱✱✱
Ankylosing spondylitis/rheumatoid arthritis. ✱✱
Infective endocarditis. ✱

This sailor had contracted gonorrhoea 15 years previously. Syphilis is often cotransmitted with this. After the primary stage, with the primary chancre at the site of inoculation associated with painless regional lymphadenitis, the secondary stage produces a generalized symmetrical rash, condylomata lata, mucosal snail-track ulcers (in the mouth or on the genitalia), painless generalized lymphadenopathy and constitutional symptoms. Many years later, tertiary syphilis may develop, manifesting itself as neurosyphilis (meningovascular syphilis, general paresis of the insane or tabes dorsalis) or as the cardiovascular form.

Cardiovascular syphilis mostly manifests itself 10–25 years following the original inoculation with *Treponema pallidum*. It may present as asymptomatic aortitis, aortic regurgitation, aortic aneurysm or coronary osteal stenosis. The chest radiograph in this patient shows evidence of aortitis and there is clinical evidence of aortic regurgitation. The angina may result from atherosclerotic coronary artery disease or from the obliterative endarteritis which causes luetic coronary osteal stenosis. This may be established at coronary angiography.

A 67-year-old man presented with pyrexia, shortness of breath, anorexia and weight loss of 1 stone over 3 months. He had a chronic cough productive of green sputum, and had suffered recurrent bouts of haemoptysis, losing a tablespoonful of fresh blood on each occasion. He had had several courses of oral antibiotics from his GP over the preceding few months.

On examination he was cachectic with a marked kyphosis. The carotid pulse was collapsing in character and his blood pressure was 110/50 mmHg. The apex beat was displaced into the sixth intercostal space, anterior axillary line and was thrusting in character. There was a 3/4 early diastolic murmur at the left sternal edge at the end of expiration. Respiratory examination showed right-sided deviation of the trachea, with reduced percussion note over the right apex. There was an increase in tactile vocal fremitus and vocal resonance, with bronchial breathing over the same area. Abdominal and neurological examination was unremarkable.

The investigations were as follows:
Hb 14 g/dl, WCC 7.1×10^9/l, Plts 244×10^9/l, ESR 26 mm/h.
Sodium 135 mmol/l, potassium 4.3 mmol/l, bicarbonate 40 mmol/l, urea 5.2 mmol/l, creatinine 75 μmol/l.
Chest radiograph: right apical shadowing, deviated trachea.

A What is the likely underlying diagnosis?

B Give the likely cause of his acute exacerbation.

C What further tests would you request?

A Ankylosing spondylitis. ✳✳✳
Aortic regurgitation. ✳

This should be apparent from the description of a man with a marked cervical kyphosis together with signs of aortic regurgitation and respiratory disease. A 'question mark' facial appearance may be apparent in an effort to ensure unobscured vision in the presence of a marked kyphosis. A clinical diagnosis can be made using Schober's test to confirm lumbar involvement and demonstrating a chest expansion of less than 5 cm to confirm costovertebral involvement. The other clue is the associated aortic regurgitation, found in up to 4% in some studies, which is as a result of a generalized aortitis. This can result in aneurysmal dilatation. Other cardiac defects include pericarditis, cardiomyopathy and cardiac conduction defects. A spinal radiograph would be expected to show squaring of the vertebrae, syndesmophyte formation causing the 'bamboo spine' appearance, erosions of the anterior-superior portion of the vertebral body (the so-called 'Romanus' lesion), fusion of the apophyseal joints and sometimes a concomitant sacroileitis.

B Tuberculosis. ✳✳
Carcinoma of the bronchus. ✳
Bronchiectasis. ✳

This man has signs consistent with right upper lobe consolidation. The 3-month history of associated signs could be consistent with tuberculous infection in this area, a region for which this organism has a predeliction. Alternatively, the right apex may have been previously damaged by fibrosis associated with the ankylosing spondylitis. Secondary infection with tuberculosis or indeed the development of bronchiectatic lung, would be more likely to occur in such an area.

C Blood cultures. ✳✳✳
Sputum microscopy, culture and cytology, screening for acid and alcohol fast bacilli (AAFB) in particular. ✳✳✳
Early morning urine for AAFB (3 samples). ✳✳
Nasogastric washings for AAFB (3 samples). ✳✳
Bronchoscopy with lavage for AAFB. ✳✳
CT chest with fine needle aspiration biopsy if a mass is seen. ✳✳
Echocardiogram. ✳

A 77-year-old man was admitted with a 2-week history of falls. He described these as his legs giving way without warning. There were no preceding palpitations or dizziness, and no evidence of fitting. Lately he complained of nausea and vomiting.

On examination his pulse was 40/min, irregularly irregular. Blood pressure was 100/60 mmHg with no postural drop. There were soft inspiratory bilateral crepitations on auscultation. The remainder of the examination was unremarkable.

Drugs on admission included:
Aspirin 75 mg o.d.
Frusemide 40 mg o.d.
Digoxin 125 μg o.d.
Captopril 25 mg b.d.
Amiodarone 200 mg o.d.

A What further tests would you request?

B Give the likely cause of his problems.

A ECG. ✱✱✱
Urea and electrolytes. ✱✱
Serum digoxin level. ✱✱
Thyroid function tests. ✱
Chest radiograph. ✱

B Amiodarone causing digitoxicity. ✱✱✱
Digitoxicity. ✱✱

This elderly patient presents in slow atrial fibrillation, with nausea and vomiting. The incidence of digoxin toxicity in the out-patient setting is said to be as high as 16% in some studies. Classically it presents with gastrointestinal symptoms, drowsiness and agitation, and disturbance of vision (xanthopsia). Cardiac manifestations of digoxin toxicity include arrhythmias, commonly coupled ventricular ectopics, but also varying degrees of atrioventricular conduction block or supraventricular dysrrhythmia (classically atrial tachycardia with 2 : 1 block). Amiodarone can increase serum digoxin levels.

A 60-year-old smoker presented with an 8-week history of colicky abdominal pain, increasing back pain, malaise and weight loss. On examination, he was afebrile, had right upper quadrant tenderness (no abdominal organomegaly) and had a palpable left supraclavicular lymph node. In addition, he had a right pleural effusion.

Initial investigations showed:
Hb 11.8 g/dl, Plts 341×10^9/l, WCC 11.7×10^9/l: neutrophils 72%, lymphocytes 9%, monocytes 9%, eosinophils 2%, basophils 1%.
Plasma viscosity 1.81.
Urea, electrolytes and calcium normal.
Albumin 27 g/l, liver function tests otherwise normal.
Thoracic and lumbar spinal views: degenerative changes only.
Chest radiograph: cardiomegaly, right pleural effusion.
Pleural aspirate: total protein 38 g/l, albumin 20 g/l, no organisms seen (including acid fast bacilli).
CT scan abdomen: Large mass of necrotic tissue encasing the aorta above and below the diaphragm. Lymphadenopathy along the lesser curve of the stomach, para-aortic area and supraclavicular fossa.

A What further investigations would you organize?

B What is the most likely diagnosis?

A Supraclavicular lymph node biopsy. ✳✳✳
CT-guided needle tissue biopsy. ✳✳✳
CT chest. ✳✳
Cytology of pleural fluid. ✳✳
CEA titre. ✳
Colonoscopy. ✳

B Lymphoma. ✳✳✳
Bronchial carcinoma with metastatic spread. ✳✳
Colonic carcinoma with metastatic spread. ✳

This patient had a non-Hodgkin's lymphoma confirmed on lymph node biopsy. The history of backache, weight loss and lymphadenopathy is suggestive of neoplasia. The abdominal CT scan is particularly helpful in making this difficult diagnosis. Ultimately, however, a histological diagnosis is essential.

A 19-year-old woman was referred to the neurologist with bizarre movements. She had been admitted 2 days earlier following a benzodiazepine overdose from which she had made a satisfactory recovery. It was on the consultant ward round that the movements were initially observed, consisting of a continuous writhing, purposeless movement of the right hand, which she controlled by using her other hand. Her right foot adopted an inverted posture. Clinical examination, including a full neurological examination, was unremarkable, her mental test score being normal.

On further questioning by the neurologist, she admitted her problems had started 4 years earlier, when she was at school. She had difficulty keeping still and had a constant desire to fidget; she found the right-hand side of her body would perform involuntary movements, which she found hard to control. Because of her fidgeting, she was regarded as a disruptive pupil by her teachers and was often asked to leave the classroom. Although excellent at her studies up to this point, she became increasingly alienated and left school at the age of 16. She became depressed over the following years and her depression was exacerbated by a miscarriage at the age of 18. She sought help for her movement disorder but this was labelled as functional secondary to her depression. She was given benzodiazepines by her GP to help with her anxiety, and took the OCP. There was no relevant family history.

A What movement disorder(s) does she manifest?

B What is the likely diagnosis?

C What investigations would you request?

A Unilateral choreo-athetosis of the right hand with right foot dystonia. ✳✳✳
Chorea. ✳✳
Dystonia. ✳

B Structural damage to the left subthalamic area caused by a space-occupying lesion or a
cerebrovascular accident. ✳✳✳
Oral contraceptive-associated chorea. ✳✳
Anti-phospholipid syndrome with associated chorea. ✳✳
Systemic lupus erythematosus with associated chorea. ✳✳
Thyrotoxicosis. ✳
Polycythaemia rubra vera. ✳
Huntington's chorea. ✳
Wilson's disease. ✳
Chorea gravidarum. ✳

C CT/MRI brain. ✳✳✳
ANA/double-stranded DNA antibody titre. ✳✳
VDRL/TPHA/antiphospholipid antibody titre/lupus anticoagulant. ✳✳
Thyroid function tests. ✳✳
ESR and CRP. ✳
Full blood count. ✳
Serum copper and caeruloplasmin. ✳
Genetic testing for Huntington's disease. ✳
Pregnancy test. ✳

Unilateral choreo-athetosis is highly suggestive of a structural disorder affecting the contralateral
subthalamic nucleus. Lesions of this area also give rise to hemi-ballismus. One should carefully screen
for anti-phospholipid syndrome (with or without associated SLE) given the history of a previous
miscarriage. Oral contraceptives and pregnancy have also been associated with chorea and
contraceptive medication should be discontinued. Huntington's chorea is unlikely given the age of
onset, the lack of a family history and the absence of dementia, but is still a possibility and may now be
screened for genetically. This particular patient turned out to have a cavernous haemangioma of the
left subthalamic nucleus.

A 34-year-old caucasian woman was admitted with a 3-week history of painless jaundice, itching, dark urine and pale stools. She had had no nausea or vomiting. She had returned from a trip to Hong Kong 3 months earlier. She admitted to half a stone in weight loss over the previous month and smoked 15 cigarettes a day. She had Hashimoto's thyroiditis diagnosed 4 years earlier, and was now on thyroxine replacement. Her mother had primary biliary cirrhosis. She had been on the OCP for many years. She was diagnosed as a Turner's mosaic, and had recently started imipramine for depression. She admitted to excessive alcohol intake in the past but denied any recent alcohol abuse.

On examination, she was icteric and apyrexial. She was very short in stature with no other obvious stigmata of Turner's syndrome. There were four spider naevi present but no other signs of chronic liver disease. The remainder of the examination was unremarkable.

Her investigations were as follows:
Hb 13.8 g/dl, total WCC 6.8×10^9/l, Plts 330×10^9/l.
Sodium 136 mmol/l, potassium 4.5 mmol/l, urea 3.6 mmol/l, creatinine 58 µmol/l, albumin 35 g/l, alkaline phosphatase 296 IU/l, bilirubin 169 µmol/l, ALT 96 IU/l.
Thyroxine 157 nmol/l, free T4 39.9 pmol/l, TSH 0.13 mU/l.
Serum IgG 6.9 g/l, serum IgA 2.01 g/l, serum IgM 0.61 g/l.
Urine analysis: negative for urobilinogen.

A What further tests would you perform?

B Give the likely diagnosis for the cause of the jaundice.

A Ultrasound of the liver. ✳✳✳
ERCP. ✳✳
Anti-mitochondrial and anti-smooth muscle antibodies. ✳✳
Serology for hepatitis A, B, C & E; EBV, CMV; HIV. ✳✳
α_1-antitrypsin level. ✳
Liver biopsy. ✳

B Jaundice secondary to imipramine/OCP combination. ✳✳✳
Associated autoimmune disease, e.g. primary biliary cirrhosis (PBC). ✳✳
HIV-associated sclerosing cholangitis. ✳
Extra-hepatic biliary obstruction, e.g. gallstones, lymphoma. ✳

The causes of obstructive jaundice may be divided into intra- and extra-hepatic types. The intra-hepatic types may be further subdivided into those with or without structural liver disease. The intra-hepatic causes without structural disease include pregnancy and the use of the OCP, benign recurrent intra-hepatic cholestasis and total perenteral nutrition (TPN). Intra-hepatic with structural disease include side-effects of drugs, e.g. chlorpromazine and erythromycin, viral hepatitides, α_1-antitrypsin deficiency, alcohol, PBC and sclerosing cholangitis. Extra-hepatic causes include any block to the hepatic ducts or the common bile duct, e.g. gallstones, carcinoma head of pancreas, cholangiocarcinoma.

The above patient has a 3-week history of an obstructive jaundice, given her pale stools and dark urine, and had returned from a trip to the Far East 3 weeks earlier. This is within the incubation period for hepatitis A, B and C. Hepatitis E has been mainly reported in the Indian subcontinent but is also a possibility here. The picture with the viral hepatitides is mainly hepatocellular but can also be obstructive. The history of the weight loss may be related to over-replacement with thyroxine but one has to consider malignancy, in this setting lymphoma (which has a higher incidence in Turner's syndrome) causing obstruction at the porta hepatis.

There is a family history of autoimmune disease and the patient herself has Hashimoto's thyroiditis. The associations of the latter are Grave's disease, pernicious anaemia, rheumatoid arthritis, Sjögren's disease, ulcerative colitis, SLE and haemolytic anaemia. PBC is made less likely by the normal IgM levels; however, it should be formally excluded with screening for the antimitochondrial antibody. Lupoid hepatitis is less likely as it gives a mainly hepatocellular picture, but unlike PBC, is directly associated with Hashimoto's thyroiditis and can be screened for by a rise in IgG and the presence of the anti-smooth muscle antibody.

The drugs are probably the likeliest culprits in this case. Both the OCP and imipramine can cause an obstructive jaundice and the former would exacerbate the effect of the latter by inhibition of hepatic enzymes.

A 27-year-old man returned from a 2-week trip to India. Prior to departure he recalled having had a full battery of immunizations including hepatitis A immunoglobulin and typhoid vaccine. He had taken regular malaria prophylaxis whilst in India but had stopped on his return. Twelve days after returning he had developed a high temperature and rigors.

On examination he was pyrexial at 38°C, and had obvious red macules on his abdomen and back. Further examination was unremarkable.

The results of his investigations were as follows:
Hb 12.5 g/dl, Plts 245×10⁹/l, WCC 6.5×10⁹/l, ESR 65 mm/h.
Thin malaria film negative.
Blood culture: Gram-negative rods in 1/3 sets.
MSU: sterile pyuria.
Chest radiograph: normal.

A What is the most likely diagnosis?

B What is the required treatment?

C What further investigations would you perform?

A Typhoid or paratyphoid fever. ✱✱✱
Viral exanthem, e.g. rubella, parvovirus or measles. ✱✱
Epstein–Barr virus (EBV). ✱✱
Cytomegalovirus (CMV). ✱✱
Malaria. ✱
Dengue fever. ✱
Urinary tract infection. ✱

B For typhoid or paratyphoid fever, an oral course of a 4-aminoquinolone, such as ciprofloxacin, is often used. One may also consider chloramphenicol, cotrimoxazole or ampicillin.

C Further malaria films, with thick films if available to increase sensitivity of detection.
Serological tests for dengue, rubella, parvovirus, measles, EBV, CMV.
Widal test for salmonella serology likely to be misleading since recently immunized.

This question is testing the candidate's ability to give a differential diagnosis for a persistent fever in the tropical traveller. In this particular case a young man, on regular antimalarial prophylaxis, develops a high temperature and macular rash centred on his thoracic wall (rose spots) following his return. He has Gram-negative rods in one set of blood cultures, which are unlikely to be a contaminant.

Salmonella, despite the lack of enteric symptoms, would explain all of the above and remains the most likely diagnosis. Typically, infection with *S. typhi* has a 10–14 day incubation period, followed by a prodrome of fairly non-specific 'flu-like' symptoms, e.g. headache and malaise. The symptoms and signs that follow are said to occur in stages. In week one, they are typically pyrexial with an inappropriate bradycardia, the erythematous maculopapular rash which blanches on pressure, is said to appear in the second week of illness, along with lymphadenopathy and hepatosplenomegaly. The third week is known as the week of complications, and here the infection can acquire a truly multi-systemic character, with lobar pneumonia, endocarditis, haemolytic anaemia, meningitis and peripheral neuropathy, acute cholecystitis and osteomyelitis (closely associated with sickle cell disease). Urinary tract infection can also occur which could explain the pyuria in this case. Typically, the infection resolves by week four.

Investigations in typhoid fever include a lymphopenia. Blood cultures give a high rate of positivity in week one. Urine and stool cultures are useful in weeks two to four. Bone marrow culture can be tried in difficult cases. Vaccination gives incomplete and short-lived protection. However, a more recent live oral vaccine, *S. typhi* (Ty21a), looks more promising.

Of the other possible diagnoses, malaria is always a possibility in the tropical traveller, despite chemoprophylaxis, as resistance to chloroquine is on the increase. *Plasmodium vivax* is the likeliest malaria to be contracted in India, and this has a much milder course than falciparum. Although this man took antimalarials whilst on holiday, he put himself at risk by not continuing them for a month on his return.

Dengue fever has a similar 'flu-like' prodrome, but has a very characteristic and transient morbilliform rash which is most pronounced in the trunk area. It gives a biphasic fever and often widespread lymphadenopathy.

The viral exanthems occur in a mainly younger age group but should not be overlooked. The distribution and form of the rash is quite characteristic in these. Koplik's spots may be present in measles and similarly Forcheimer spots of the soft palate in rubella. The macular rash is mainly facial and becomes characteristically confluent and discoloured in measles.

EBV and CMV can both present with a 'flu-like' illness and a macular rash. There is often a mild hepatitis present and jaundice can occur.

A 65-year-old retired primary school teacher was seen in the out-patients' clinic complaining of an 18-month history of increasing shortness of breath on exertion and swelling of her ankles. The problem had started gradually and was not preceded by chest pain. She had no orthopnoea or paroxysmal nocturnal dyspnoea. She had lost half a stone in weight. She smoked heavily and kept no pets. Her GP had started her on diuretics.

On examination she was short of breath with a dusky red discoloration of her cheeks and over her nose. There was no clubbing. The jugular venous pressure (JVP) was raised to the earlobes and 'cv' waves were seen. The apex was displaced. Heart sounds were normal with a soft pansystolic murmur at the left sternal edge, which did not radiate. There was pitting oedema to the knees bilaterally. Respiratory examination revealed fine bibasal inspiratory crepitations not cleared on coughing. Abdominal examination revealed a two-finger breadth pulsatile liver edge.

The results of her investigations were as follows:
Hb 12.9 g/dL, total WCC 8.1×10^9/l, Plts 342×10^9/l.
ESR 8 mm/h, C-reactive protein 6 mg/l.
Sodium 137 mmol/l, potassium 4.9 mmol/l, bicarbonate 31 mmol/l, urea 8.8 mmol/l, creatinine 112 µmol/l, albumin 32 g/l, alkaline phosphatase 107 IU/l, total bilirubin 35 µmol/l, ALT 50 IU/l, calcium 2.55 mmol/l (corrected value 2.7 mmol/l), phosphate 1.3 mmol/l.

A Give a possible diagnostic test.

B What further tests would you perform?

C What is the likeliest underlying diagnosis?

D How would you manage this patient?

A Bronchoalveolar lavage. ✳✳✳
Liver biopsy. ✳✳
The Kveim test was previously widely used in the diagnosis of sarcoidosis. The material was homogenized human spleen from patients who had died from sarcoidosis. This material cannot be certified free of HIV and this test is no longer available.

B Chest radiograph. ✳✳✳
Gallium scan. ✳✳
Arterial blood gases. ✳✳
Serum angiotensin converting enzyme (ACE) level. ✳✳
Respiratory function tests: FEV_1, FVC and TLCO. ✳✳
Echocardiography. ✳

C Sarcoidosis. ✳✳✳
Pulmonary hypertension secondary to fibrotic lung disease. ✳

D Steroids are the mainstay of treatment and may produce resolution of the primary disease as well as correcting the hypercalcaemia.

This patient has a gradual onset of mainly right-sided heart failure with functional tricuspid regurgitation, secondary to primary lung pathology given the bibasal crepitations in the absence of a history of orthopnoea or paroxysmal nocturnal dyspnoea (PND). Cryptogenic fibrosing alveolitis is unlikely due to the absence of clubbing. The dusky discoloration of the cheeks and nose is due to lupus pernio. Although this may superficially resemble the characteristic facial appearance seen in association with SLE, the normal ESR and age of the patient make this unlikely. Sarcoidosis presents in over 30-year-olds as a chronic disease with lupus pernio and pulmonary infiltrates (rather than erythema nodosum and bi-hilar lymphadenopathy).
Serum ACE is raised in approximately 70% of active disease cases. Bronchoscopy can occasionally reveal sarcoid deposits in the bronchial tree and lavage will show a lymphocytic infiltrate with a reduced IgG level. Lung function reveals an increased FEV_1/FVC with a reduced TLCO.
The corrected calcium in this case was calculated as follows:

correction factor $= (40\,g/l - \text{albumin concentration in } g/l) \times 0.02$, i.e. $(40 - 32) \times 0.02 = 0.16$

corrected calcium $= 2.55\,mmol/l + 0.16\,mmol/l = 2.71\,mmol/l$

The granulomata in sarcoidosis can express 1 α-hydroxylase and therefore activate vitamin D inappropriately, causing hypercalcaemia in the presence of normal serum phosphate levels.

A 74-year-old man with known nephrotic syndrome, normally managed at a nearby specialist renal centre, was admitted with a 2-week history of increasing swelling of his legs and a 2-day history of increasing shortness of breath. He had known chronic obstructive airways disease (COAD) and had had polio as a child.

On admission he was on 280 mg of frusemide and 15 mg of amiloride a day. He had a temperature of 37.8°C. His heart rate was 130/min with a blood pressure of 170/110 mmHg and the JVP was at the level of his ear lobes. The apex was not displaced and there was a 2/6 pansystolic murmur at the left sternal edge, which did not radiate. His respiratory rate was 20/min and auscultation revealed bibasal inspiratory crepitations and marked expiratory wheeze. There was pitting oedema to the sacrum.

The following investigations were obtained:
Hb 12.6 g/dl, total WCC 15×10^9/l, Plts 333×10^9/l.
Clotting studies normal.
Sodium 137 mmol/l, potassium 4.4 mmol/l, bicarbonate 23 mmol/l, urea 14.2 mmol/l, creatinine 214 μmol/l, albumin 19 g/l, alkaline phosphatase 59 IU/l, ALT 24 IU/l.
Urine dipstick: protein +++, blood +++.
Chest radiograph: hyper-expanded chest with upper lobe diversion, Kerley B lines and fluid in the horizontal fissures.

A What is the likely cause of his acute deterioration?

He was treated with intravenous antibiotics and high-dose intravenous diuretics. He initially made good progress but a few days later his renal function deteriorated further and his potassium became elevated to 6.3 mmol/l with a urea of 26 mmol/l and a creatinine of 280 μmol/l. He complained of left loin pain and became anuric.

B What is the likeliest cause of his further deterioration?

C What would be your further management?

A Urinary tract infection. *******
Infective exacerbation of COAD. ******
Pulmonary emboli. *****

Patients with nephrotic syndrome are very susceptible to infection, particularly *Pneumococcus*, which may cause spontaneous bacterial peritonitis in the presence of ascites. This is partly due to the low levels of IgG in this condition; additionally, it is thought that products of the alternative complement pathway are lost in the urine. Some advocate prophylactic penicillin for all nephrotic patients for this reason.

B Acute renal vein thrombosis. *******
Over diuresis causing acute on chronic renal failure. *****

Renal vein thrombosis classically presents with loin pain, acute renal failure and haematuria. It is said to occur in up to 50% of nephrotics in some studies, and is also said to be commoner in nephrotic syndrome associated with underlying amyloidosis, membranous and mesangiocapillary glomerulonephritis. It occurs in the setting of hypercoagulability of the blood due to loss of antithrombin III and proteins C & S in the urine, together with increased platelets and fibrinogen. Diagnosis is made by Doppler ultrasonography.

C Control of potassium with insulin/dextrose. *******
Urgent ultrasound examination to exclude renal vein thrombosis. ******
Anti-coagulation if necessary. ******
Central line insertion and fluid challenge if appropriate — salt poor albumin is ideal for this purpose as it mobilizes the peripheral oedema. *****

A 43-year-old man was admitted with a 1-week history of watery diarrhoea, abdominal pain, haematemesis and abdominal swelling. He had suffered a series of recent chest infections for which he had sought the advice of his GP. He was a known alcoholic and intravenous drug abuser. He was taking erythromycin and frusemide on admission.

On examination he was icteric and pyrexial. There were spider naevi, scratch marks and a liver flap present. Abdominal examination revealed a four-finger breadth, tender, liver edge, a palpable spleen and ascites. There was marked constructional apraxia.

His initial investigations are shown:
Hb 9.5 g/d, total WCC 4.4×10^9/l, Plts 22×10^9/l.
PT 22 s, APTT 52 s, fibrinogen 3.4 g/l.

Sodium 133 mmol/l, potassium 1.9 mmol/l, bicarbonate 25 mmol/l, urea 1.6 mmol/l, creatinine 61 µmol/l, albumin 24 g/l, alkaline phosphatase 176 IU/l, ALT 19 IU/l, bilirubin 73 µmol/l.

A What is the likely cause of the thrombocytopenia?

B What are the possible causes of his deterioration?

C What further tests would you request?

D How would you manage this patient?

E Why is he hypokalaemic?

A Hypersplenism. ✱✱✱
Disseminated intravascular coagulation (DIC). ✱
The differential diagnosis of decreased platelets with increased APTT and PT is:
- liver disease with hypersplenism
- DIC — less likely in this case as the fibrinogen is not reduced
- chronic heparin treatment

B Intercurrent infection, e.g. spontaneous bacterial peritonitis, chest infection. ✱✱✱
Diarrhoea causing dehydration and metabolic abnormality. ✱✱
Erythromycin treatment causing obstructive jaundice. ✱✱
Recent alcohol binge. ✱
Haematemesis. ✱

C Chest radiograph. ✱✱✱
Blood cultures. ✱✱✱
Mid-stream specimen of urine (MSU). ✱✱✱
Ascitic tap sent for biochemistry, microscopy with Gram stain, and culture. ✱✱✱
Stool culture and analysis for *Clostridium difficile* toxin. ✱✱
Assessment of encephalopathy with 'five-pointed star' chart, plasma ammonia level and EEG. ✱✱
Endoscopy. ✱

D Treat intercurrent sepsis. ✱✱✱
Correct metabolic abnormality: withdraw diuretics and alcohol. ✱✱
Stop erythromycin. ✱✱
Treat gastrointestinal bleed if found on endoscopy. ✱✱
Lactulose to acidify the gut and convert ammonia to NH_4^+ ions. ✱✱
Gut sterilization with neomycin enema. ✱
Treatment of coagulation defects with FFP, platelets and vitamin K. ✱
Thiamine supplementation. ✱

E Secondary hyperaldosteronism. ✱✱✱
Frusemide. ✱

Hypoalbuminaemia causes secondary hyperaldosteronism. This in turn causes hypokalaemia. Thus frusemide is an inappropriate diuretic: spironalactone (an aldosterone receptor antagonist) would be more appropriate. Chronic therapy with either spironalactone or amiloride may, however, cause gynaecomastia. At presentation the total body potassium is usually very low and patients may require over 500 mmol KCl before the potassium normalizes.

A 62-year-old man presented with a 2-day history of projectile vomiting. He admitted to a 1-month history of weight loss with loss of appetite. He was a heavy smoker who was otherwise fit. Physical examination revealed marked cachexia with a non-pulsatile, fixed epigastric mass on abdominal palpation.

A What is the likely diagnosis?

B What electrolyte/acid–base abnormalities would you expect to find and why?

A Pyloric stenosis secondary to adenocarcinoma of the stomach. ✳✳✳
Pyloric stenosis. ✳✳
Adenocarcinoma of the stomach. ✳
Pancreatic tumour. ✳

B Hypochloraemic, hypokalaemic, metabolic alkalosis with a raised urea. ✳✳✳
Hypochloraemic, hypokalaemic, metabolic alkalosis. ✳✳

Vomiting accompanying pyloric stenosis leads to loss of hydrogen and chloride ions from the stomach contents. The dehydration caused by the profuse vomiting leads to a fall in glomerular filtration rate which in turn leads to a decrease in renal excretion of bicarbonate. Due to the loss of chloride ions, sodium uptake from the distal convoluted tubule is made possible by one-to-one exchange for either hydrogen ions, worsening the alkalosis, or potassium ions leading to hypokalaemia.

A 53-year-old farmer presented with a 3-week history of drenching night sweats and a temperature. He complained of weakness, lethargy and weight loss. His GP had prescribed him a course of antibiotics, but due to the nausea induced by the medication, his compliance had been poor. Two days prior to admission, his testicles had become swollen and painful. He was a South African who had emigrated to the UK 5 years previously. He had visited his homeland a month earlier. His past medical history included tuberculosis, malaria and hypertension. He was taking antihypertensive medication only.

On examination he was pyrexial with a temperature of 38°C. Shotty cervical lymph nodes were present. Blood pressure was 160/100 mmHg. The cardiac apex was displaced and thrusting and there was a 3/6 ejection systolic murmur over the aortic area and a 2/4 early diastolic murmur at the fourth intercostal space, left sternal edge. Respiratory examination revealed bibasal inspiratory crepitations, and in the abdomen there was a two-finger breadth liver with a palpable spleen tip. The testicles were mildly swollen and were obviously inflamed and tender.

The results of the investigations are as follows:
Hb 11.1 g/dl, MCV 84 fl, Plts 180×10^9/l, WCC 6.8×10^9/l: neutrophils 1.0, lymphocytes 5.0, monocytes 0.7, eosinophils 0.1.
Blood film report: relative lymphocytosis with atypical lymphocytes; no malarial parasites seen.
Sodium 130 mmol/l, potassium 4.3 mmol/l, urea 3.2 mmol/l, creatinine 115 μmol/l, albumin 36 g/l, ALT 90 IU/l, alkaline phosphatase 140 IU/l, bilirubin 17 μmol/l.
ESR 130 mm/h, CRP 240 mg/l.
Chest radiograph: right apical fibrosis; fluid in the horizontal fissure; upper lobe blood diversion; right pleural effusion.

A   What is the likely diagnosis for this man's underlying condition?

B   What further tests would you perform?

A Brucellosis. ✱✱✱
Bacterial endocarditis. ✱✱
Tuberculosis. ✱
Reactivation or recent acquisition of malaria. ✱

B Blood cultures. ✱✱✱
Brucella serology. ✱✱✱
Echocardiography. ✱✱
Further malaria films. ✱✱
Pleural biopsy for granulomata. ✱✱
Sputum/early morning urine/nasopharyngeal aspirate or broncho-alveolar lavage for auramine/Ziehl–Nielsen staining for AAFB. ✱
Bone marrow culture. ✱

Brucella is a Gram-negative coccobacillus which has been largely eliminated from cattle in the UK. It is commonly acquired through the ingestion of unpasteurized milk and invades the lymph nodes and reticulo-endothelial system via the lymphatics. The incubation period is up to 3 weeks and the onset is often insidious, resulting in the classical undulant fever pattern. Lymphadenopathy, hepatosplenomegaly, arthritis and back pain, endocarditis, orchitis and meningoencephalitis can all follow. Blood cultures in the acute phase of infection are positive in 50% and a 4-fold rise over a 4-week period, or a single titre of 1 : 60, in the *Brucella* agglutination test is highly suggestive of infection.

A 60-year-old man presented with severe abdominal pain. There was evidence of a profuse rectal bleed. No history was available from the patient. His daughter stated that her father had been previously fit until the last 2 months when he had begun to suffer from episodes of fainting. He was on no medication.

After fluid resuscitation, his blood pressure was 110/95 mmHg and he was mildly pyrexial. His cardiac apex was not displaced and was heaving in nature. There was a 4/6 ejection systolic murmur heard at the left sternal edge and over the aortic area, which radiated to both carotids. There was, in addition, a 2/4 early diastolic murmur, heard best at the fourth intercostal space, left sternal edge, in held end expiration. Respiratory examination revealed bibasal inspiratory crepitations. The abdomen was soft and non-tender and rectal examination revealed an empty rectum with the presence of fresh blood.

The results of his investigations were as follows:
Hb 11.5 g/dl, MCV 72 fl, Plts 290 × 10^9/l, ESR 55 mm/h.

Sodium 134 mmol/l, potassium 4.8 mmol/l, urea 5.8 mmol/l, creatinine 110 µmol/l.

A Give the likely unifying diagnosis for the above presentation.

B What further investigations would you request?

A Mixed aortic valve disease with angiodysplasia. ✳✳✳
Subacute bacterial endocarditis causing mixed aortic valve disease with emboli causing ischaemic colitis. ✳✳

B Blood cultures. ✳✳✳
Echocardiography. ✳✳
Colonoscopy. ✳✳
Selective mesenteric angiography. ✳
Urine dipstick for haematuria. ✳
Double contrast barium enema. ✳

Angiodysplasia has an increasing incidence in the older age group and has an association with aortic stenosis. There is often a past medical history of recurrent gastrointestinal bleeds of unknown origin. Localization of the bleeding vessel may be made by selective mesenteric angiography or by direct visualization on colonoscopy. Treatment is by colonoscopic fulguration of the involved vessels.

Ischaemic colitis usually presents with left-sided iliac fossa pain and loose motions containing fresh blood. The mucosa appears blue on colonoscopy and contrast barium enema shows 'thumb-printing' of the affected bowel.

A 31-year-old housewife was referred by her GP to the medical team on-call. She gave a 2-day history of frontal headaches, vomiting and backache. She had been seen by her doctor 2 days previously and was prescribed a course of penicillin for a presumed chest infection. A left cerebello-pontine angle tumour had been removed 2 years previously, with an episode of post-operative meningitis. Ten months following this, a ventriculo-peritoneal shunt was inserted for hydrocephalus.

On examination, her temperature was 37.8°C. A left posterior craniotomy defect was palpable with no apparent bulging of this area. Fundoscopy was normal. Her pupils were equal and reacting to light and she had a left lower motor neurone VII nerve palsy. Kernig's sign was positive and there was increased cervical tone. Her physical examination was otherwise unremarkable.

Initial investigations were as follows:
Hb 10.9 g/dl, WCC 9.9×10^9/l, Plts 297×10^9/l.

A What is the most likely diagnosis?

B What investigations would you perform immediately?

C What treatment would you institute?

A Bacterial meningitis due to shunt infection. ✳✳✳
Recurrence of left cerebello-pontine angle tumour with malignant meningitis. ✳✳
Recurrence of left cerebello-pontine angle tumour. ✳
Obstruction of ventriculo-peritoneal shunt. ✳

B MRI brain. ✳✳✳
Lumbar puncture. ✳✳✳
CT scan of the brain. ✳✳
Blood cultures. ✳

C Antibiotic therapy, analgesia and anti-emetic therapy. Ultimate eradication of the infection may involve removal and replacement of the shunt.

In a patient presenting in this manner, who has undergone several neurosurgical procedures and has a ventriculo-peritoneal shunt *in situ*, the diagnosis of bacterial meningitis is the most likely possibility. Given the presence of a ventriculo-peritoneal shunt, obstruction of this will also need to be excluded. The histology of the original tumour is not given in the question, and recurrence of tumour with possible malignant meningitis must also be considered.

Since she has already had several days of penicillin therapy, she is likely to have a partially treated meningitis. It is therefore unlikely that a CSF gram stain will reveal any organisms; the detection of bacterial antigens in the CSF may be more helpful.

The commonest organisms causing bacterial meningitis in adults are *Streptococcus pneumoniae* (<50% cases), followed by *Neisseria meningitidis* (<35% cases) and *Haemophilus influenzae*, type B (<3% cases). Meningitis following neurosurgical procedures, particularly shunt insertion, tends to involve a different group of organisms: *Staphylococcus epidermidis* (which causes 75% of all infections associated with shunting procedures with hydrocephalus), *Staphylococcus aureus* and Gram-negative bacilli, e.g. *Escherichia coli*, *Proteus*, *Klebsiella* and *Pseudomonas*. The usual blind treatment of bacterial meningitis is with cefotaxime.

Listing by specialty

Index

Numbers are page numbers, *not* case numbers.